Abteilung für Medizinische Psychologie
Direktorin: Prof. Dr. rer. biol. hum. N. von Steinbüchel
Georg-August-Universität Göttingen
Waldweg 37
37073 Göttingen

D1731194

The Assessment of Cognitive Function in Epilepsy

EDITORS

W. Edwin Dodson, M.D.
Washington University, School of Medicine
St. Louis, Missouri

Marcel Kinsbourne, M.D.
Sargent College, Boston University
Boston, Massachusetts

Beat Hiltbrunner, M.D.
Medical Department, Ciba-Geigy Ltd
Basel, Switzerland

Demos Publications, 386 Park Avenue South, Suite 201, New York, New York 10016

Acknowledgment

The workshop on which this volume was based was organized under the auspices of the Behavioral Sciences Initiative Group of the Continuing and Professional Education Committee of the Epilepsy Foundation of America, supported by a grant from the Ciba-Geigy Corporation in Basel, Switzerland. Its objectives reflect the desire of the Epilepsy Foundation of America to stimulate research into the cognitive and behavioral difficulties that affect some people with epilepsy.

Manufactured in the United States of America

Great care has been taken to maintain the accuracy of the information contained in this volume. However, neither the editors nor Demos Publications can be held responsible for errors or for any consequences arising from the use of the information contained herein.

Editorial, Design, & Composition by
Roberta J. Landi Book Production, Old Saybrook, Connecticut

ISBN: 0-000-000-000-X

Contents

Preface

Patients with epilepsy have a threefold greater risk of cognitive and other mental problems than individuals without neurologic problems. The factors that contribute to this increased risk include the direct effects of seizures, the effects of associated (usually antecedent) neuropsychological deficits, and adverse medication effects. Further, more than half of patients with epilepsy first develop seizures in childhood. For these reasons, computerized assessment of specific cognitive functions in patients with epilepsy presents both special problems and special opportunities.

The need to characterize the various approaches to automated or computerized assessment of neuropsychological functions was emphasized at the International Epilepsy Meeting in New Delhi, India, in October of 1989, at which several investigators described various effects of seizures and antiepileptic drugs on cognitive functions in patients with epilepsy. In most cases, the cognitive functions were measured by automated or computerized tasks designed to assess particular mental functions. Although each group of investigators used computerized assessments with unique features, their approaches overlapped due to the sharing of computerized applications by workers in the field. For this reason, the origins of computerized tasks, as well as the specifics of the tasks used by various workers, needs to be defined both for clarification currently and with a view toward eventual standardization.

On the basis of this need, a workshop titled "Assessing Cognitive Function in Patients with Epilepsy" was held in Bermuda in March of 1991; the current volume presents the results of this meeting. Its objective was to define existing computerized testing methods with respect to those being applied to the assessment of neuropsychological functions in patients with epilepsy. Particular emphasis was placed on the role of computerized testing in monitoring cognitive effects of antiepileptic agents in patients of varying ages. The relevance, validity, and reliability of the various approaches were also addressed. Although many investigators are exploring computerized neuropsychological testing, the participants at this workshop are leaders in applying these techniques to persons with a variety of disorders—especially epilepsy. The workshop did not deal with the details of computerized scoring or with the interpretation of traditional tests that evaluate global neuropsychological functioning.

The genealogy of automated and computerized testing in epilepsy provides some insight into the relationships of the various approaches used by different investigators. FePsy—the iron psychologist—is the most comprehensive and widely used system for computerized assessment of specific neuropsychological functions. This system, developed at the Instituut voor Epilepsiebestrijding at Heemstede in the Netherlands, has been nurtured by Dr. Bert Aldenkamp and Dr. Willem Alpherts, who (in 1978) began work on this system under the supervision of D. van Zijl. Initially written in FORTRAN and Z80 assembler for the Zilog 80 computer, the programs were subsequently adapted for the Apple II-E. In 1987, the programs were converted to MSDOS, based on Turbo-Pascal, and in 1990 this system was updated for 80386-based personal computers with VGA color graphics and a built-in interface to combine EEG registration with computerized testing.

FePsy has affected the approaches taken by others. Dr. Pamela Thompson developed tasks in her own laboratory that were later adapted for the investigations of drug effects done by Dr. Thompson and Dr. Michael Trimble; these in turn were shared with Dr. Carl Dodrill. Currently, Thompson and her group use a combination of FePsy and her original test battery. Subsequently, Dodrill has developed a novel series of automated tasks that are altogether different from FePsy items. Separately, an adaptation of the Corsi Block test was developed by Dr. Colin Binnie at Meer en Bosch to assess the effects of epileptic discharges on cognitive functions. A similar version is also represented in FePsy, both for stand-alone testing procedures and for combining neuropsychological testing and EEG registration.

Other investigators, who developed their testing methodologies independently, often interacted with the group at Heemstede. For example, Dr. Anna-Lise Rugland in Norway developed a computer game as a continuous performance task. This task can be integrated with EEG data to determine the effect of epileptic discharges as well as the effect of drugs on overall performance. It is planned to merge Rugland's computer game and EEG interfaces into FePsy and vice versa. Binnie's adaptation of the Corsi Block test is part of the Rugland battery.

Other investigators have developed computerized approaches without interacting with the Heemstede group; this applies to certain tests for children. For example, continuous performance and learning tasks for the Apple Macintosh computer were developed by Dr. Marcel Kinsbourne for quantitating the cognitive gains conferred by stimulant drug therapy in children with attention deficit–hyperactivity disorders. He has also developed tests of impulsivity and organization. The automated tests developed by Dr. Michael Aman also focus on the assessment of drug effects in children, but have both a different lineage and the special property of being applicable to children with mental retardation.

One of the several tasks in Dr. Aman's system is based on the Sternberg model-based test of short-term memory that Dr. Keith Scott developed at the University of Illinois for evaluating mentally retarded children. In the 1970s, Dr. Robert Sprague adapted this and other tasks for studies of stimulant medications in children. Working in New Zealand in the 1980s, Dr. Aman and Dr. John Werry extended the array of tasks into an automated motor performance battery. Initially constructed from relays and switches, this system eventually became personal computer based. The system utilizes a unique set of ingenious peripheral devices that are described in this volume; thus far, Dr. Aman's system has not been used by others.

Although much work remains to be done before the computerized assessment of specific cognitive functions is perfected and standardized, this approach has already produced important insights and holds great promise for the future. Pending chores include the development of tasks that are applicable to a broader range of ages and mental abilities, and the need for systematic determination of the validity and reliability of various tasks. Notwithstanding, these approaches already save time and are greeted by high patient acceptance when applied appropriately. It must be emphasized, however, that these are not replacements for traditional neuropsychological evaluation. These increase, rather than reduce, the need for neuropsychological expertise in dealing with patients with complex cognitive and behavioral problems.

Computerized techniques for measuring neuropsychological functions have far-reaching implications for disorders other than epilepsy. Computerized assessment of specific mental functions is relevant wherever disease or drugs have the potential to affect mental functioning.

The workshop on which this volume is based was organized under the auspices of the Behavioral Sciences Initiative Group of the Continuing and Professional Education Committee of the Epilepsy Foundation of America, supported by a grant from the Ciba-Geigy Corporation in Basel, Switzerland. Its objectives reflect the desire of the Epilepsy Foundation of America to stimulate research into the cognitive and behavioral difficulties that affect some people with epilepsy.

W. Edwin Dodson, M.D.
St. Louis, Missouri, U.S.A.

Marcel Kinsbourne, M.D.
Boston, Massachusetts, U.S.A.

Beat Hiltbrunner, M.D.

Contributors

A.P. Aldenkamp—Instituut voor Epilepsiebestrijding 'Meer & Bosch/De Cruquiushoeve', Heemstede, The Netherlands

W.C.J. Alpherts—Instituut voor Epilepsiebestrijding 'Meer & Bosch/De Cruquiushoeve', Heemstede, The Netherlands

Michael G. Aman—The Nisonger Center for Mental Retardation and Developmental Disabilities, The Ohio State University

C.D. Binnie—Maudsley Hospital, London, England

H. Bjørnæs—National Center for Epilepsy, Sandvika, Norway

Carl B. Dodrill—Regional Epilepsy Center, University of Washington School of Medicine, Seattle, Washington

W. Edwin Dodson—Washington University, School of Medicine, St. Louis, Missouri

O. Henriksen—The National Center for Epilepsy, Sandvika, Norway

Bruce P. Hermann—Epi Care Center, Baptist Memorial Hospital; Departments of Psychiatry and Neurosurgery, University of Tennessee, Memphis; Semmes–Murphy Clinic, Memphis, Tennessee

Beat Hiltbrunner—Medical Department, Ciba-Geigy Limited, Basel, Switzerland

Tony Johnson—Medical Research Council Biostatistics Unit, Cambridge, United Kingdom

Marcel Kinsbourne—Behavioral Neurology Unit, Sargent College of Allied Health Professions, Boston, Massachusetts

M.D. Lezak—Department of Neurology, School of Medicine, Oregon Health Sciences University

J. Overweg—Instituut voor Epilepsiebestrijding 'Meer & Bosch/De Cruquiushoeve', Heemstede, The Netherlands

Ernst Pöppel—Institut für medizinische Psychologie, Ludwig-Maximilians-Universität München

A-L. Rugland—The National Center for Epilepsy, Sandvika, Norway

Pamela J. Thompson—Epilepsy Research Group, National Hospitals, Chalfont Centre for Epilepsy, London, England

J.A.P. Van Parijs—Instituut voor Epilepsiebestrijding 'Meer & Bosch/De Cruquiushoeve', Heemstede, The Netherlands

N.P.L.G. Verhoeff—Academic Medical Centre, Department of Nuclear Medicine, Amsterdam, The Netherlands

J. Vermeulen—Instituut voor Epilepsiebestrijding 'Meer & Bosch/De Cruquiushoeve', Heemstede, The Netherlands

Nicole von Steinbüchel—Institut für medizinische Psychologie, Ludwig-Maximilians-Universität München

1

Contributions of Traditional Assessment Procedures to an Understanding of the Neuropsychology of Epilepsy

Bruce P. Hermann, Ph.D.

Epi Care Center, Baptist Memorial Hospital
Departments of Psychiatry and Neurosurgery, University of Tennessee, Memphis
Semmes-Murphey Clinic, Memphis, Tennessee

Introduction

Interest is growing in the use of computerized neuropsychological techniques to define the effects of epilepsy and its treatments on higher cognitive functions. This interest follows the development of a very rich and extensive literature on the neuropsychological correlates of the epilepsies, a literature that has relied almost exclusively on traditional methods of assessment. This literature serves as the basis upon which information from the new technology will be compared and its value decided. Familiarity with the structure of this literature is therefore important. The purpose of this chapter is to identify the major research interests, trends, and contributions evident in the neuropsychological research that has been published during this century. Several themes will be reviewed, placed in an historical context, and briefly illustrated.

Traditional assessment essentially refers to the administration of conventional tests of intelligence, achievement, and/or measures of discrete cognitive functions (e.g., memory, visual perception, language). Many of these tests have been

TABLE 1

Themes of Neuropsychological Research in the 1900s

1. Intelligence and cognitive deterioration in epilepsy
2. Neuroseizure variables (e.g., seizure type, etiology, age at onset, duration of disorder) and cognitive function
3. Effects of EEG abnormalities (e.g., nature and frequency of EEG abnormalities) on neuropsychological function
4. Epilepsy surgery and neuropsychological status
5. Investigations into the tests themselves
6. Ability of neuropsychological tests to help resolve difficult clinical issues (pseudoseizures, psychopathology)
7. Childhood epilepsy and cognitive status and academic achievement
8. Anticonvulsant medications and cognitive abilities

well standardized on large normative populations, others are more experimental in nature and have been derived for special purposes. The use of these procedures has resulted in its share of highlights and lowlights, insights and gross miscalculations. Overall, however, with the kind cooperation of literally thousands of willing persons with epilepsy who have endured the imposition of a bevy of psychologists and psychometricians, the effects of epilepsy on higher cognitive functions have been characterized with increasing precision.

Before beginning, one caveat needs to be made. This is not a critical review of the intellectual and neuropsychological effects of epilepsy. Excellent reviews of this topic are available elsewhere (Bennett & Krien 1989; Dikmen 1980; Dodrill 1988; Folsom 1952; Keating 1960; Tarter 1972). Rather, this presentation is intended to serve as a brief historical overview of neuropsychological research in this century, highlighting several of the major themes of cognitive assessment in epilepsy that relied almost exclusively on traditional (noncomputerized) assessment procedures but are now increasingly the subject of computerized evaluation.

If one scans the neuropsychological and cognitive literature that has been published during this century, several major overall themes and research interests are evident (Table 1). An overall sense of the progress, limitations, and contributions of traditional assessment methodologies will be presented here using the framework of Table 1 while at the same time the opportunities for the newer computerized technologies in these areas will be considered.

Intelligence and Cognitive Deterioration in Epilepsy

The history of cognitive assessment in epilepsy has paralleled developments in the broader field of psychometrics. For example, Binet's approach to the assessment of intelligence (Binet–Simon Scales of 1905, 1908, and 1911), and the modification of these procedures for use in the United States (Stanford–Binet Test developed by Terman in 1916) attracted a considerable amount of attention in the psychological community (Anastasi 1969). It did not take long for these tests to be applied to persons with epilepsy with the first published uses appearing prior to 1920.

Most of the earlier investigations sought merely to describe the intellectual status of patients with epilepsy by providing mean IQ scores. These reports demonstrated interest in the notion that cognitive deterioration occurred in a substantial proportion of patients. However, one very early investigation (Fox 1924) was quite sophisticated for its time, and anticipated many of the research trends that would become evident during the next six to seven decades.

J. Tylor Fox (1924) examined patients with epilepsy who were residents in a special facility—the Lingfield Epileptic Colony in the U.K. It is of some historical note to mention that the 150 children in this study (age 5–16 years) met the criteria specified in the so-called Defective and Epileptic Children Act of 1889. Those criteria specified that a qualified practitioner, approved by the Board of Education, certified that the child was not retarded, but was unfit to attend an ordinary public elementary school because of frequent or severe epilepsy. Not surprisingly, the median IQ scores (Binet–Simon Test) of these children was relatively depressed (boys = 71, girls = 65).

However, Fox also administered tests of reading, spelling, arithmetic, and reasoning, as well as the Porteus Mazes—a still-popular neuropsychological measure. This report, therefore, represents one of the first attempts to quantitate the academic achievement of a group of children with epilepsy. Their achievement scores were lower than normal and in some cases even lower than would be predicted given their IQ, making this report one of the first demonstrations of academic underachievement among children with intractable epilepsy. Fox also retested a large sample of the children (N = 130) one year later. He reported wide variations in test–retest performance with, as was stressed, a general tendency to deterioration and with very marked deterioration in over 8%.

Fox appreciated and commented on the variability in psychometric performance that was evident among the patients, and speculated that variables such as seizure type, seizure severity, or etiological considerations might account for this performance variability and should be the subject of future investigations. As will become evident, such attempts did indeed occupy a considerable proportion of the subsequent neuropsychological literature.

The relationship between epilepsy and cognitive deterioration remained of interest for some time. Publications concerned with cognitive deterioration appeared in the 1920s (Dawson & Conn 1929; Patterson & Fonner 1928), 1930s (Paskind 1932; Barnes & Fetterman 1938; Fetterman & Barnes 1934), 1940s (Arieff & Yacorzynski 1942; Hilkevitch 1946; Yacorzynski & Arieff 1942), 1950s (Davies-Eysenck 1952), and even up to the 1980s (Bourgrois et al. 1983; Trimble 1984). Arguments were put forward both for (Dawson & Conn 1929; Fox 1924) and against the concept (Barnes & Fetterman 1938; Fetterman & Barnes 1934; Hilkevitch 1946; Patterson & Fonner 1928); see Keating (1960) for a review up to 1960. Others suggested that deterioration appeared only in certain subgroups of patients with epilepsy, for instance, only among those with a certain underlying etiology (Arieff & Yacorzynski 1942; Yacorzynski & Arieff 1942). Clarification of the presence/absence of deterioration, and the frequency with which it occurred, was confounded by variations in the definition of deterioration. Some authors referred to deterioration in the sense that it would be used today: a progressive *loss* of intellectual ability over time. But others used it in reference to a relative *decrement* of intellectual abilities compared to controls (Folsom 1952).

Patients continued to be studied at selected sites such as colonies, hospital dispensaries, state hospitals, and other specialized facilities. Tarter reviewed the literature in 1972 and summarized 17 studies published between 1924 to 1968 that utilized various measures of intelligence (Binet-Simon, Stanford-Binet, Binet-Burt, Progressive Matrices, Wechsler-Bellevue [WAIS, WISC]). Whereas more than half of the investigations (9 of 17) were carried out with institutionalized individuals, not surprisingly, an overrepresentation of below average IQ scores was found. The special nature of groups such as these was eventually noted by some investigators, particularly Lennox (1942), who felt them to be unrepresentative of the general population of persons with epilepsy. Indeed, in a large-scale investigation Collins and Lennox (1947) reported that among their private patients, the mean IQ of 100 children with epilepsy (Stanford-Binet Form L) was 104. The mean IQ of 200 adults with epilepsy (Wechsler-Bellevue) was 111.

The essential lesson taught by Lennox and reiterated some years later by Folsom (1952), was generally not appreciated by subsequent epilepsy researchers. The fact that groups of *patients* with epilepsy are available for research at selected sites, and the fact that quantitative research may be carried out at those sites, does not mean that the results are generalizable to *all persons* with epilepsy. The most recent example of this lesson is in the field of research concerned with the relationship between epilepsy and psychopathology. Rates of psychopathology noted in selected samples of patients presenting to specialized epilepsy centers, surgical series, university hospitals and the like do not generalize to community groups of persons with epilepsy (Edeh et al. 1990; Trostle et al. 1989; Zielinski 1986)—a point raised by Janice Stevens some years ago (Stevens 1975).

Interest in the possibility of cognitive deterioration associated with ongoing epilepsy has continued up to the present. Trimble (1984) recently noted "that some patients with epilepsy undergo a deterioration of their cognitive abilities is clear from clinical experience." Investigating 40 patients with epilepsy at the Chalfont Center for Epilepsy, performance on a modified Wechsler Adult

Intelligence Scale (WAIS) was compared to estimated premorbid IQ. When deterioration was defined as a drop of over 15 IQ points, 21 of the 40 patients had deteriorated. Deterioration was significantly associated with widening of the sulci of the cerebellum and vermis, generalized tonic-clonic seizures, head injuries, and total intake of phenytoin and primidone.

In a very sophisticated prospective study of children with epilepsy (Bourgrois et al. 1983) it was found that deteriorating IQ was associated with an earlier age at onset, poorer seizure control, greater total number of seizures, greater number of drugs taken simultaneously, increased incidence of toxic drug levels, and increased number of different drugs for which toxic levels were found.

Additional research has identified the adverse intellectual and psychosocial consequences associated with increasing lifetime numbers of generalized tonic-clonic seizures (Dodrill 1986).

Neuroseizure Variables and Cognitive Function

The hypothesis raised by Fox in 1942 that a variety of variables such as seizure type, severity, and etiology might bear a relationship to the adequacy of intellectual function, has been amply borne out during the subsequent seven decades. The effects of these and other relevant variables have been examined on intelligence tests, neuropsychological batteries, and measures of discrete cognitive abilities. A few examples illustrate the point.

Collins and Lennox's (1947) important work again serves as an example. Examining mean IQ scores in 100 children (Stanford–Binet) and 200 adults (Wechsler–Bellevue) with epilepsy, they found that a symptomatic etiology (presence of an acquired brain lesion) played a significant role in both groups. The IQ of the symptomatic groups was approximately 10 points lower. When examining the role of seizure type, they found that the highest IQ values were associated with petit mal epilepsy and the lowest were associated with having both grand mal and psychomotor seizures. IQ scores were also found to be associated with particular EEG patterns, a point which will be discussed later.

A more contemporary and elegant demonstration of the effects of seizure variables on intelligence and neuropsychological function was provided by Matthews and Klove (1967). They examined groups of patients with major motor, psychomotor, and mixed seizures of known and unknown etiology, as well as control groups of both patients with brain damage without seizures and non-neurological patients on the WAIS and Halsted tests (Table 2). The results indicated regularities in findings as a function of seizure type and etiology. In general, patients with symptomatic epilepsy performed more poorly than those with idiopathic epilepsy; those with psychomotor seizures performed better than those with major motor or mixed seizure types. Interestingly, patients with idiopathic psychomotor seizures of unknown etiology were quite comparable to the non-neurological patients. A large number of additional investigations have

TABLE 2

Impairment Index Ratings for Eight Groups

Rating	Groups	Mean Impairment Index*
Best	1. Non-neurological	3.22
	2. Psychomotor seizures of unknown etiology	3.45
	3. Psychomotor seizures of known etiology	5.45
	4. Mixed (major motor and psychomotor) of unknown etiology	5.78
	5. Major motor seizures of unknown etiology	5.83
	6. Mixed (major motor and psychomotor) of known etiology	6.30
	7. Verified brain damage without epilepsy	7.19
Worst	8. Major motor seizures of known etiology	7.48

Notes: Modified from Matthews and Klove (1967). *Number of tests outside of normal limits.

examined the effects of seizure type, age at onset of epilepsy, laterality of seizure foci, and other variables on general neuropsychological batteries (e.g., Dikmen et al. 1975, 1977; Dikmen & Matthews 1977; Klove & Matthews 1966; O'Leary et al. 1981, 1983).

Finally, the effects of diverse seizure-related variables have been examined on a variety of discrete cognitive abilities. A prime example is memory (Delaney et al. 1980; Lee et al. 1989; Loring et al. 1989; Mungas et al. 1985; Sass et al. 1990; Tucker et al. 1986).

The essential point is that considerable diversity exists in the adequacy of cognitive function among patients with epilepsy. Lennox was very interested in this diversity and discussed what he called the "five foes of mental competence." These include genetic influences, organic abnormalities of the brain acquired prior to the onset of the epilepsy, the epilepsy itself and the pathological sequelae of seizures, psychosocial isolation, and overdose with sedative anticonvulsants (Lennox & Lennox 1960). Certainly these and other factors influence the diversity of cognitive status in epilepsy. The ability of computerized assessment procedures to identify other variables of influence will be of considerable interest.

Effects of EEG Abnormalities on Neuropsychological Function

Epileptiform neuronal discharges are a defining feature of epilepsy. These abnormal discharges can vary in frequency, pattern, amplitude, and other characteristics. During the early part of this century considerable efforts were devoted to identifying the EEG correlates of a variety of clinical seizure types. For instance, the 3 Hz spike-wave pattern associated with petit mal epilepsy was described by Gibbs and collaborators in 1935. In 1937 the association between "square-shaped waves" and so-called psychomotor seizures was reported for the first time (Gibbs et al. 1937). After these important discoveries investigators soon began to inquire into the effects of such abnormal discharges on neuropsychological functions.

In 1939 Schwab published one of the first investigations of the effects of spike-wave discharges on cognitive performance. This initiated one major branch of the neuropsychology-EEG literature, one that has been concerned with the effects of "subclinical" petit mal discharges on tasks of cognitive ability. Tests used for this purpose include the Continuous Performance Test (CPT) (Mirsky & Van Buren 1965), pursuit-rotor task (Goode et al. 1970), decision-making measures and other tests (Tizard & Margerison 1963).

As an example of this literature, Mirsky and Van Buren (1965) compared patients with centrencephalic (absence or petit mal) seizures with those with epilepsy of focal origin on the CPT, a test of sustained attention and vigilance. Patients with absence seizures were found to be more impaired on the X task of the CPT. During subclinical spike-wave bursts the patients averaged 24% correct responses, while in the absence of bursts the patients performed correctly on 85% of the trials. A fuller account of the impairing effects of subclinical spike-wave discharges on cognitive functions can be found in Mirsky's recent review (1989).

A second branch of the neuropsychology-EEG literature has examined the effects of a variety of abnormal EEG characteristics such as frequency, distribution, and rate of abnormal discharges on various qualitative and quantitative neuropsychological indices (Dodrill & Wilkus 1976a; Hovey & Kooi 1955; Klove 1959; Klove & White 1963; Parsons & Kemp 1960; Pihl 1968; Wilkus & Dodrill 1976). A few examples reflect the scope of interest in this area.

Hovey and Kooi (1955) studied the relationship between "nonanswer responses," or NRs (responses which indicated a momentary deviation from an established goal idea), and patients' performances on the Wechsler intelligence tests. NRs essentially represented *qualitative* abnormalities in test performance. For instance, on a given subtest of the WAIS a patient might be providing appropriate and correct answers, but then may suddenly make a careless error or appear as if not engaged in the task at hand, only to subsequently resume his or her previously appropriate performance. Three groups (epilepsy, brain damage without epilepsy, psychiatric patients) were studied using the Wechsler–Bellevue. A higher proportion of patients with epilepsy manifested NRs (44%) compared to the organic (17%) and psychiatric patients (9%). The implication was that abnormal psychometric test performance, transient and qualitative in nature, could be the result of abnormal EEG activity. This point was later confirmed during simultaneous EEG and psychological testing (Kooi & Hoovey 1957).

Dodrill and Wilkus (1976a) examined EEG effects further and studied the influence of the presence, average rate, and topographic distribution of discharges on WAIS performance. Lower intelligence levels were associated with the presence of discharges, especially when generalized rather than focal, and with discharge rates of more than one per minute. Additional work by these investigators demonstrated the effects of such discharges on Halsted–Reitan performance (Wilkus & Dodrill 1976), and the relationship between other abnormal EEG patterns and neuropsychological performance (e.g., Dodrill & Wilkus 1976b).

Similar impairing effects of epileptiform activity on neuropsychological performance have been detected when interictal EEG recordings have been obtained using depth electrodes (Rausch et al. 1978). Given the expansion of surgical epilepsy centers and the accompanying use of intracranial EEG procedures, further investigation in this field is expected.

This important field of investigation has been pursued via computerized methodology (Shewmon & Erwin 1988a,b,c). Some have suggested that the term *transient cognitive impairment* be used to refer to the impairing effects of interictal epileptiform discharges (Aarts et al. 1984; Binnie et al. 1987).

Epilepsy Surgery and Neuropsychological Status

In 1939 Donald Hebb reported on a patient who had undergone right temporal lobectomy for treatment of intractable epilepsy. Hebb drew a careful distinction between the effects of such surgery on intelligence compared to more discrete cognitive abilities. He noted that the patient's good postoperative IQ score was not evidence that other cognitive abilities were spared, and he suggested that normal intelligence was a complex concept whose components could be differentiated by cerebral lesions. The patient retained good language skills (e.g., Thorndike Word Knowledge, Kelley–Trabue Language Completion) but had a concomitant disturbance of nonlanguage capacities including form perception, visual and nonvisual, and disturbance of social comprehension (e.g., Knox Cube, Seguin, Feature Profile) (Hebb 1939).

The following year Hebb and Penfield (1940) presented the results of psychological assessment following frontal lobectomy and suggested that removal of a chronically discharging lesion might be less disruptive to an individual's cognitive abilities than its presence. Hebbs' early provocative papers might be viewed as the beginning of a very close association between neuropsychology and epilepsy surgery. Indeed, from the Montreal Neurological Institute came the seminal studies of Brenda Milner and her collaborators. These have yielded a wealth of understanding of brain-behavior relationships in general, and of the hippocampal model of memory function in particular (Milner 1958, 1972, 1975, 1986).

Bailey and Gibbs at the University of Illinois in Chicago, established a new era in epilepsy surgery in 1947 by operating on patients who had intractable epilepsy, but who did not have an underlying structural lesion. That is, patients were selected for surgery on the basis of interictal EEG criteria in association with the fact that the epilepsy had strong adverse effects on their lives (Bailey & Gibbs 1951). From the outset, the group at Illinois was concerned with the effects of surgery on the patients' neuropsychological status and behavioral and emotional adjustment. Bailey enlisted the help of Ward Halsted, just across town at the University of Chicago, to study his patients following anterior temporal lobectomy (Hermann & Stone 1989). Halsted, using his now widely known battery of neuropsychological tests, concluded that following anterior temporal lobectomy there was an improvement on most neuropsychological indicators, but that performance was still impaired in relation to normal controls. At the very least, he could detect no severe deficits attributable to surgical intervention. Further neuropsychological studies from the psychologists at Illinois extended these findings (Simmel & Counts 1958).

As epilepsy surgery developed and expanded, so did the role of neuropsychological investigation. As Taylor (1979) noted, psychological testing has been used in at least four ways:

1. to facilitate an understanding of the cerebral organization of verbal and visuospatial skills of the patients;

2. to help identify the area of epileptogenicity and related areas where brain dysfunction exists;

3. to identify the risks of surgery to essential psychological functions such as speech, memory, and other important functions; and

4. to provide some prognosis as to the effects of the epilepsy surgery (e.g., Bengzon et al. 1968; Wannamaker & Matthews 1976).

To that list should be added the role of neuropsychology in assessing the outcome of epilepsy surgery.

Important findings quickly emerged from the first generation groups, such as Milner and her collaborators at the Montreal Neurological Institute (Milner 1986), Lansdell at the National Institutes of Health (Lansdell 1968a,b), and Meyer at the Maudsley Hospital (Meyer & Yates 1955; Meyer 1959). Neuropsychological assessment has remained an important clinical and research component at virtually all surgical epilepsy centers.

Investigations of the Tests Themselves

As the number and diversity of neuropsychological tests proliferated, more specific questions were asked, and more demands were placed on the tests. In many instances the tests themselves became the objects of investigation. At least three trends can be identified in the literature.

First, several studies have examined the ability of specific tests or test batteries to identify the presence of "organic impairment of cognitive function" associated with epilepsy. For instance, the ability of the Luria–Nebraska Neuropsychological Battery to identify the presence of organic impairment of cognitive functions has been undertaken with mixed results (Berg & Golden 1981; Hermann & Melyn 1985; Moses et al. 1988). More fruitful efforts were demonstrated by Dodrill, who modified the Halsted–Reitan battery in order to improve its sensitivity to cognitive impairment in epilepsy. On cross-validation his modified battery (Neuropsychological Battery for Epilepsy) was found to identify 84% of normals and 72% of epilepsy patients (Dodrill 1978).

The utility of individual tests has been similarly investigated. Examples include the Canter Background interference procedure for the Bender Gestalt test, and the Trail Making test (Delaney 1982; McKinzey et al. 1985). Such efforts have generally been unsuccessful because the "hit rate" in such cases is often unacceptably low, as noted by Delaney (1982).

Second, several investigations have attempted to derive test indices that discriminate patients with varying seizure types, most commonly seeking to differentiate temporal lobe epilepsy from primary generalized epilepsies. This has been attempted with the Wechsler intelligence tests with mixed results (Bolter et al. 1981; Milberg et al. 1980), the Continuous Performance Test on which patients with absence seizures have been found to perform more poorly (Lansdell & Mirsky 1964), or to identify a measure sensitive to particular subgroups of patients with temporal lobe epilepsy, for instance those with right temporal lobe damage (Kimura 1963; Shalman 1961).

Third, several investigations have examined issues of psychometric interest among patients with epilepsy, such as the distribution of VIQ–PIQ splits and factors that influence either the frequency or magnitude of such splits (e.g., gender, EEG factors) (Dennerll 1964a; Dennerll et al. 1964b; Fowler et al. 1980; Lin 1979; Parsons & Kemp 1960), the factor structure of the Wechsler tests among patients with epilepsy and their similarity/dissimilarity to normative groups (Dennerll et al. 1964b; Fowler et al. 1980), or the problems posed by *repeated* testing with neuropsychological instruments (Dodrill & Troupin 1975; Seidenberg et al. 1981b).

Greater understanding of the psychometric characteristics of the tests themselves, and consideration of the demographic and other (nonepilepsy related) factors that influence their variability, will help to differentiate the signal from noise in such test measurements.

Ability of Neuropsychological Tests to Help Resolve Difficult Clinical Issues

A more recent development has concerned the use of traditional neuropsychological assessment to help in the management of difficult diagnostic issues, the monitoring of treatment efficacy, or evaluation of the contribution of neuropsychological impairment to important psychosocial problems. Several examples can be provided.

1.   The diagnostic problems involved in discriminating pseudoseizures from actual seizures are widely appreciated, and the ability of neuropsychological tests and measures to aid in this discrimination have been studied (Sackellares et al. 1985; Wilkus et al. 1984). While neuropsychological tests and emotional/behavioral measures do not appear to be of singular diagnostic significance, these do appear to provide information that will assist in this most difficult diagnostic problem when used in conjunction with other neurological and psychiatrical findings.

2.   The difficulties faced by individuals with epilepsy in the workforce are well known. At least some of the employment difficulties may be attributable to cognitive impairment associated with the patients' epilepsy, or to its underlying etiology. Several investigations identified features of cognition that are associated with employment difficulties (Dennerll et al. 1966; Dikmen & Morgan 1980; Schwartz et al. 1968). The ability of neuropsychological tests to predict future employment problems has proven promising (Dodrill & Clemmons 1984).

3.   Emotional and behavioral problems among patients with epilepsy are a difficult management issue. The causes of such problems are likely multifactorial encompassing neurological, psychosocial, and iatrogenic issues (Hermann & Whitman 1984). Neuropsychological factors, such as the overall adequacy of higher cognitive functions or particular patterns of deficits, may be associated with psychiatric difficulties (Camfield et al. 1984; Csernansky et al. 1990; Hermann 1982), but not all evidence supports this view (Moehele et al. 1984).

4.   Assessment of neuropsychological abilities may help monitor the effects of anticonvulsant medications or changes in the patients' clinical status. For instance, the beneficial effects of improved seizure control on cognitive status, or the alteration of anticonvulsant management regimens such as reduction of barbiturate medications have been demonstrated with traditional neuropsychological tests (Davies-Eysenck 1952; Giordani et al. 1983; Seidenberg et al. 1981a).

5.   As has been alluded to above, traditional assessment measures have been used to monitor the effects of epilepsy surgery on patients' quality of life. Measures of general intellectual ability (Meier & French 1966) as well as discrete cognitive functions such as language (Hermann & Wyler 1988; Lifrak & Novelly 1984; Stafiniak et al. 1990), memory (Katz et al. 1989; Meyer & Jones 1957; Milner 1968; Novelly et al. 1984; Rausch & Babb 1987), and other abilities may help make it possible to modify surgical techniques in order to provide the best surgical outcome with the least associated neuropsychological morbidity.

Childhood Epilepsy and Cognitive Status and Academic Achievement

One of the cruel ironies of epilepsy is that it very frequently makes its appearance in childhood, a time of crucial neurocognitive development and a period when a variety of important skills and abilities are being acquired. Children with epilepsy, and the status of their neuropsychological functions, have been the subject of continuing interest since Fox's early quantitative report (Keating 1960; Seidenberg 1989a,b). Many of the themes discussed thus far (such as lower IQ in institutionalized individuals and lower IQ associated with symptomatic etiology) have also been noted repeatedly in children. Several relatively specific research themes and interests can be identified in the pediatric epilepsy literature.

1. Children and adolescents have been studied not only with standard intelligence tests, but also with more sophisticated batteries of neuropsychological tests (e.g., Reitan-Indiana Battery) and with various combinations of specialized measures (Camfield et al. 1984; Dean 1983; Farwell et al. 1985; O'Leary et al. 1981, 1983). For instance, Farwell et al. (1985) compared 118 children with epilepsy with 100 controls, all subjects were between 6–15 years old, on the WISC-R and age-appropriate Halsted–Reitan tests. Children with epilepsy had lower intelligence levels—except for those with classic absence only. Intelligence was also related to the degree of seizure control. On the neuropsychological tests, the children with epilepsy were similarly more impaired than were the controls.

2. Issues of academic achievement continue to be investigated with standardized measures such as the Wide Range Achievement Test. Again, children with epilepsy appear at heightened risk of academic underachievement in

TABLE 3

Academic Underachievement Among Children with Epilepsy*

Variables	Percent Significantly Underachieving	
	Males (N = 54)	Females (N = 68)
Word recognition	10.5	10.1
Spelling	33.3	15.9
Arithmetic	28.1	31.9
Reading comprehension	22.8	13.0

Notes: Modified from Seidenberg (1989a). *Children were classified as significant underachievers if their obtained academic score was one standard deviation below their expected score based on a WISC-R Full Scale IQ level.

reading, spelling, reading comprehension, mathematics ability (Camfield et al. 1984; Farwell et al. 1985; Green & Hartlage 1971; Rutter et al. 1970; Seidenberg et al. 1986; Stores 1976), as well as in more general indices of school progress (Holdsworth & Whitmore 1974; Pazzaglia & Frank-Pazzaglia 1976). Table 3 provides a summary of the proportion of children with epilepsy attending a specialized epilepsy center and the degree of academic under-achievement adjusted for expectations based on IQ levels.

3. Contemporary research has examined the role of factors such as laterality of temporal lobe focus, seizure type, and other demographic and neuroseizure variables (e.g., age at onset) in placing children at risk for discrete impairments in cognitive function, academic underachievement, and impairments in neuro-psychological performance (Camfield et al. 1984; Fedio & Mirsky 1967; O'Leary et al. 1981, 1983; Stores 1976).

While this work would seem to be subject to the sorts of selection biases that were noted earlier, the epidemiological work of Rutter and his colleagues in the Isle of Wight study suggest that even among a general population, childhood epilepsy carries with it some hazard to learning and achievement (Rutter et al. 1970).

The particular risk to academic and general life adjustment associated with impairment of language skills has been highlighted by several groups. Seidenberg et al. (1987) found evidence that language impairment was associated with particular risk for academic underachievement. Dodrill and Clemmons (1984) found that language difficulties earlier in life were associated with later psychosocial difficulties.

Anticonvulsant Medications and Neuropsychological Function

This has become a very active field of research, with at least 15 published reviews of the literature (Dodrill 1988). With so many reviews available, little need be said here. The use of computerized neuropsychological assessment in the evaluation of anticonvulsant medications is a major topic of this volume. Therefore, the comments offered here concern only major issues.

Just to appreciate the complexity of this literature, note that Dodrill was able to locate 78 studies of the cognitive effects of antiepilepsy medications. These investigations varied widely in their experimental design (Table 4). Clearly, evaluation of the effects of anticonvulsant medications has occupied a signifi-cant proportion of neuropsychological research.

The many reviews and large number of empirical studies reflect widespread concern about the effects of antiepilepsy medications. This concern is not new. Strenuous arguments over many issues has proceeded apace. For example,

TABLE 4

Design of 78 Studies of the Cognitive Effects of Antiepileptic Drugs

I. Studies of patients with epilepsy (N = 40)

    A. Cross-sectional (N = 8)
      1. Single agents (N = 2)
      2. Multiple agents (N = 6)

    B. Longitudinal (N = 32)
      1. With systematic drug changes (N = 29)
        a. Single agents (N = 20)
          (1) Crossover designs (N = 7)
          (2) Add-on studies (N = 5)
          (3) Untreated patients (N = 8)
        b. Multiple agents, multiple drug changes (N = 3)
      2. Without systematic drug changes (N = 3)

II. Studies of subjects without epilepsy (N = 38)

    A. Single active agents versus placebo (N = 38)
      1. Benzodiazepines (N = 18)
      2. Phenytoin (N = 8)
      3. Barbiturates (N = 7)
      4. Valproic acid (N = 3)
      5. Succinimides (N = 2)

Note: From C.B. Dodrill (1988).

bromides were both widely attacked and staunchly defended (Yacorzynski & Arieff 1942; Paskind 1934). Phenobarbital has been an object of concern for some time, though various studies demonstrated no impairing effect (Somerfeld-Ziskind & Ziskind 1940; Wapner et al. 1962), as well as significant adverse effects (Hutt et al. 1968; MacLeod et al. 1978). Most anticonvulsant drugs now undergo stringent cognitive evaluation, or comparative study (e.g., ethosuximide in Browne et al. 1975; sodium valproate in Trimble & Thompson 1984; carbamazepine in Andrewes et al. 1986; Dodrill & Troupin 1977; Schain et al. 1977; and phenytoin in Dodrill 1975; Thompson 1983).

Heated arguments continue regarding the effects of anticonvulsant medications. This debate is healthy, as it reflects widespread concern regarding the effects of treatment on the quality of life. One of the challenges will be to determine when psychometric changes are of clinical significance.

Conclusions

A rich heritage and extensive database characterize the field of neuropsychological assessment of patients with epilepsy. This field, until recently, relied on traditional methods of assessment. These methods are often slow, tedious, labor-intensive, redundant, and expensive. In the wrong hands they have been terribly stigmatizing. But, their overall yield has been impressive.

Although computerized neuropsychological assessment is relatively new, its application to epilepsy offers considerable potential. It promises sophisticated, efficient, lower cost assessment characterized by exquisite precision. How this technology will actually alter our understanding of the neuropsychological consequences of epilepsy remains to be seen. Supersensitive measurement techniques may simply lead to a bevy of *statistically* significant findings of uncertain *clinical* significance, or may result in important shifts in our understanding of the consequences of the epilepsies. Time will tell whether computerized assessment will merely replicate with greater precision what is known, or will lead to new insights in our understanding of epilepsy.

References

Aarts JHP, Binnie CD, Smit AM & Wilkins AJ. Selective cognitive impairment during focal and generalized epileptiform EEG activity. *Brain*, 1984, 107:293-308.

Anastasi A. (1969). *Psychological testing.* Toronto: Macmillan Co.

Andrewes DG, Bullen JG, Tomlinson L, Elwes RDC & Reynolds EH. A comparative study of the cognitive effects of phenytoin and carbamazepine in new referrals with epilepsy. *Epilepsia*, 1986, 27:128-134.

Arieff A & Yacorzynski GK. Deterioration of patients with organic epilepsy. *J Nerv Ment Dis*, 1942, 96:49-55.

Bailey P & Gibbs FA. The surgical treatment of psychomotor epilepsy. *J Am Med Assoc*, 1951, 145:365-370.

Barnes MR & Fetterman JL. Mentality of dispensary epileptic patients. *Arch Neurol Psychiatry*, 1938, 40:903-910.

Bengzon ARA, Rasmussen T, Gloor P et al. Prognostic factors in the surgical treatment of temporal lobe epileptics. *Neurology*, 1968, 18:717-731.

Bennett TL & Krien LK. (1989). The neuropsychology of epilepsy: Psychological and social impact. In: CR Reynolds & E Fletcher-Janzen (eds.), *Handbook of clinical child neuropsychology.* New York: Plenum Press.

Berg RA & Golden CJ. Identification of neuropsychological deficits in epilepsy using the Luria-Nebraska Neuropsychological Battery. *J Consult Clin Psychol*, 1981, 49:745-747.

Binnie CD, Kastelejin-Nolst Trente D, Smit AM, & Wilkins AJ. Interactions of epileptiform EEG discharges and cognition. *Epilepsy Res*, 1987, 1:239-245.

Bolter J, Veneklasen J & Long CJ. Investigation of WAIS effectiveness in discriminating between temporal and generalized seizure patients. *J Consult Clin Psychol*, 1981, 49:549-553.

Bourgrois BFD, Prensky AL, Palkes HS, Talent BK & Busch GB. Intelligence in children: A prospective study in children. *Ann Neurol*, 1983, 14:438-444.

Browne TR, Dreifuss FE, Dyken PR, Goode DJ, Penry JK, Porter RJ, White BG & White PT. Ethosuximide in the treatment of absence (petit mal) seizures. *Neurology*, 1975, 25:515-524.

Camfield PE, Gates R, Rosen G, Camfield C, Fergueson A & McDonald GW. Comparison of cognitive ability, personality profile, and school success in epileptic children with pure right versus left temporal lobe EEG foci. *Ann Neurol*, 1984, 15:122-126.

Collins AL & Lennox WG. The intelligence of 300 private epileptic patients. *Assoc Res Nerv Men Dis*, 1947, 26:586-603.

Csernansky JG, Leiderman DB, Mandabach M & Moses JA. Psychopathology and limbic epilepsy: Relationship to seizure variables and neuropsychological function. *Epilepsia*, 1990, 31:275-280.

Davies-Eysenck M. Cognitive factors in epilepsy. *J Neurol Neurosurg Psychiatry*, 1952, 15:39-44.

Dawson S & Conn JCM. The intelligence of epileptic children. *Arch Dis of Childhood*, 1929, 4:142-151.

Dean RS. Neuropsychological correlates of total seizures with major motor epileptic children. *Clin Neuropsychology*, 1983, 5:1-3.

Delaney RC. Screening for organicity: The problem of subtle neuropsychological deficit and diagnosis. *J Clin Psychol*, 1982, 38:843-846.

Delaney RC, Rosen AJ, Mattson RH & Novelly RA. Memory function in focal epilepsy: A comparison of non-surgical, unilateral temporal lobe and frontal lobe samples. *Cortex*, 1980, 16:103-117.

Dennerll RD. Prediction of unilateral brain dysfunction using Wechsler test scores. *J Consult Psychol*, 1964a, 28:278-284.

Dennerll RD, den Broeder J & Sokolov S. WISC and WAIS factors in children and adults with epilepsy. *J Clin Psychol*, 1964b, 20:236-240.

Dennerll RD, Rodin EA, Gonzalez S, Schwartz ML & Lin Y. Neurological and psychological factors related to employability of persons with epilepsy. *Epilepsia*, 1966, 7:318-329.

Dikmen S. (1980). Neuropsychological aspects of epilepsy. In: BP Hermann (ed.), *A multidisciplinary handbook of epilepsy* (pp. 36-73). Springfield, IL: Charles C. Thomas.

Dikmen S & Matthews CG. Effect of major motor seizure frequency upon cognitive-intellectual functions in adults. *Epilepsia*, 1977, 18:21-29.

Dikmen S, Matthews CG & Harley JP. The effect of early versus late onset of major motor epilepsy upon cognitive-intellectual performance. *Epilepsia*, 1975, 16: 73-81.

Dikmen S, Matthews CG & Harley JP. Effect of early versus late onset of major motor epilepsy on cognitive-intellectual performance: Further considerations. *Epilepsia*, 1977, 18:31-36.

Dikmen S & Morgan SF. Neuropsychological factors related to employability and occupational status in persons with epilepsy. *J Nerv Ment Dis*, 1980, 168: 236-240.

Dodrill CB. Diphenylhydantoin serum levels, toxicity, and neuropsychological performance in patients with epilepsy. *Epilepsia*, 1975, 16:593-600.

Dodrill C. A neuropsychological battery for epilepsy. *Epilepsia*, 1978, 19:611-623.

Dodrill C. Correlates of generalized tonic-clonic seizures with intellectual, neuropsychological, emotional, and social function in patients with epilepsy. *Epilepsia*, 1986, 27:399-411.

Dodrill C. (1988). Neuropsychology. In: J Laidlaw, A Richens, & J Oxley (eds.), *A textbook of epilepsy*. New York: Churchill Livingstone.

Dodrill CB. Effects of anticonvulsant drugs on abilities. *J Clin Psychiatry*, 1988, 49 (Suppl):31-34.

Dodrill C & Clemmons D. Use of neuropsychological tests to identify high school students with epilepsy who later demonstrate inadequate performances in life. *J Consult Clin Psychol*, 1984, 52:520-527.

Dodrill CB & Troupin AS. Effects of repeated administrations of a comprehensive neuropsychological battery among chronic epileptics. *J Nerv Ment Dis*, 1975, 161:185-190.

Dodrill CB & Troupin AS. Psychotropic effects of carbamazepine in epilepsy: A double-blind comparison with phenytoin. *Neurology*, 1977, 27: 1023-1028.

Dodrill C & Wilkus RJ. Relationships between intelligence and electroencephalographic epileptiform activity in adult epileptics. *Neurology*, 1976a, 26:525-531.

Dodrill C & Wilkus RJ. Neuropsychological correlates of the electroencephalogram in epileptics: II. The waking posterior rhythm and its interaction with epileptiform activity. *Epilepsia*, 1976b, 17:101-109.

Edeh J, Toone BK & Corney RH. Epilepsy, psychiatric morbidity, and social dysfunction in general practice: Comparison between hospital clinic patients and clinic nonattenders. *Neuropsychiatry, Neuropsychol, Behav Neurol*, 1990, 3:180-192.

Farwell JR, Dodrill C & Batzel LW. Neuropsychological abilities of children with epilepsy. *Epilepsia*, 1985, 26:395-400.

Fedio P & Mirsky AF. Selective intellectual deficits in children with temporal lobe or centrencephalic epilepsy. *Neuropsychologia*, 1967, 7:287-300.

Fetterman JL & Barnes MR. Serial studies of the intelligence of patients with epilepsy. *Arch Neurol Psychiatry*, 1934, 32:797.

Folsom A. Psychological testing in epilepsy. I. Cognitive function. *Epilepsia*, 1952, 1:15-22.

Fowler PC, Richards HC & Boll TJ. WAIS factor patterns of epileptic and normal adults. *J Clin Neuropsychol*, 1980, 2:115-123.

Fox JT. The response of epileptic children to mental and educational tests. *Brit J Med Psychol*, 1924, 4:235-248.

Gibbs FA, Davis H & Lennox WG. The electro-encephalogram in epilepsy and in conditions of impaired consciousness. *Arch Neurol Psych*, 1935, 34:1133-1148.

Gibbs FA, Gibbs EL & Lennox WG. Epilepsy: A paroxysmal cerebral dysrhythmia. *Brain*, 1937, 60:377-388.

Giordani B, Sackellares JC, Miller S, Berent S, Sutula T, Seidenberg M, Boll TJ, O'Leary D & Dreifuss FE. Improvement in neuropsychological performance in patients with refractory seizures after intensive diagnostic and therapeutic intervention. *Neurology*, 1983, 33:489-493.

Goode DJ, Penry JK & Dreifuss FE. Effects of paroxysmal spike-wave activity on continuous visual-motor performance. *Epilepsia*, 1970, 11:241-254.

Green JB & Hartlage LC. Comparative performance of epileptic and nonepileptic children and adults (on tests of academic, communicative and social skills). *Dis Nerv Sys*, 1971, 32:418-421.

Hebb DO. Intelligence in man after large removals of cerebral tissue: Defects following right temporal lobectomy. *J Gen Psychol*, 1939, 21:437-446.

Hebb DO & Penfield W. Human behavior after extensive bilateral removal from the frontal lobes. *Arch Neurol Psychiatry*, 1940, 44:421-438.

Hermann BP. Neuropsychological functioning and psychopathology in children with epilepsy. *Epilepsia*, 1982, 23:545-554.

Hermann BP & Melyn M. Identification of neuropsychological deficits in epilepsy using the Luria-Nebraska Neuropsychological Battery: A replication attempt. *J Clin Exp Neuropsychol*, 1985, 7:305-313.

Hermann BP & Stone JL. A historical review of the epilepsy surgery program at the University of Illinois Medical Center: The contributions of Bailey, Gibbs, and collaborators to the refinement of anterior temporal lobectomy. *J Epilepsy*, 1989, 2:155-163.

Hermann BP & Whitman S. Behavioral and personality correlates of epilepsy: A review, methodological critique and conceptual model. *Psychol Bulletin*, 1984, 95:451-497.

Hermann BP & Wyler AR. Effects of anterior temporal lobectomy on language function: A controlled study. *Ann Neurol*, 1988, 23:585-588.

Hilkevitch RR. A study of the intelligence of institutionalized epileptics of the idopathic type. *J Orthopsychiatry*, 1946, 16:262-270.

Holdsworth L & Whitmore K. A study of children with epilepsy attending ordinary schools: Their seizure patterns, progress and behavior in school. *Dev Med Child Neurol*, 1974, 16:746-758.

Hovey HB & Kooi KA. Transient disturbances of thought processes and epilepsy. *Arch Neurol Psychiatry*, 1955, 74:287-292.

Hutt SJ, Jackson PM, Belsham A & Higgins G. Perceptual-motor behaviour in relation to blood phenobarbitone level: A preliminary report. *Dev Med Child Neurol*, 1968, 10:626-632.

Katz A, Awad IA, Kong AK, Chelune GJ, Naugle R, Wyllie E, Beauchamp G & Luders H. Extent of resection in temporal lobectomy for epilepsy. II. Memory changes and neurologic complications. *Epilepsia*, 1989, 30:763-771.

Keating LE. A review of the literature on the relationship of epilepsy and intelligence in school children. *J Ment Sci*, 1960, 106:1042-1059.

Kimura D. Right temporal lobe damage. *Arch Neurol*, 1963, 8:48-55.

Klove H. Relationship of differential electroencephalographic patterns to distribution of Wechsler-Bellevue scores. *Neurology*, 1959, 9:871-876.

Klove H & Matthews CG. Psychometric and adaptive abilities in epilepsy with differential etiology. *Epilepsia*, 1966, 7:330-338.

Klove H & White PT. The relationship of electroencephalographic abnormality to the distribution of Wechsler-Bellevue scores. *Neurology*, 1963, 13:423-400.

Kooi KA & Hovey HB. Alterations in mental function and paroxysmal cerebral activity. *Arch Neurol Psychiatry*, 1957, 78:264-271.

Lansdell H. Effect of extent of temporal lobe ablations on two lateralized deficits. *Physiol Behav*, 1968a, 3:271-273.

Lansdell H. The use of factor scores from the Wechsler-Bellevue scale of intelligence in assessing patients with temporal lobe removals. *Cortex*, 1968b, 4:257-268.

Lansdell H & Mirsky AF. Attention in focal and centrencephalic epilepsy. *Exp Neurol*, 1964, 9:463-469.

Lee GP, Loring DW & Thompson JL. Construct validity of material-specific memory measures following unilateral temporal lobectomy. *Psychol Assess*, 1989, 1:192-197.

Lennox WG. Mental defect in epilepsy and the influence of heredity. *Am J Psychiatry*, 1942, 98:733-739.

Lennox W & Lennox M. (1960). *Epilepsy and related disorders* (vols. 1 and 2). Boston: Little, Brown and Co.

Lifrak MD & Novelly RA. (1984). Language deficits in patients with temporal lobectomy for complex partial seizures. In: RJ Porter et al. (eds.), *Advances in neurology: XVth Epilepsy International Symposium* (pp. 469-473). New York: Raven Press.

Lin Y. Note on WAIS verbal-performance differences in IQ. *Percep Motor Skills*, 1979, 49:888-890.

Loring DW, Lee GP, Martin RC & Meador KJ. Verbal and visual memory index discrepancies from the Wechsler Memory Scale-Revised: Cautions in interpretation. *Psychol Assess*, 1989, 1:198-202.

MacLeod CM, Dekaban AS & Hunt E. Memory impairment in epileptic patients: Selective effects of phenobarbital concentration. *Science*, 1978, 202:1102-1104.

Matthews CG & Klove H. Differential psychological performances in major motor, psychomotor, and mixed seizure classifications of known and unknown etiology. *Epilepsia*, 1967, 8:117-128.

McKinzey RK, Curley JF & Fish JM. False negatives, Canter's background interference procedure, the Trail Making test, and epileptics. *J Clin Psychol*, 1985, 41:812-820.

Meier MJ & French LA. Longitudinal assessment of intellectual functioning following unilateral temporal lobectomy. *J Clin Psychol*, 1966, 22:22-27.

Meyer V. Cognitive changes following temporal lobectomy for relief of temporal lobe epilepsy. *Arch Neurol Psychiatry*, 1959, 81:299-309.

Meyer V & Jones HG. Patterns of cognitive test performance as functions of the lateral localization of cerebral abnormalities in the temporal lobe. *J Ment Sci*, 1957, 103:758-772.

Meyer V & Yates AJ. Intellectual changes following temporal lobectomy for psychomotor epilepsy: Preliminary communication. *J Neurol Neurosurg Psychiatry*, 1955, 18:44-52.

Milberg W, Greiffenstein M, Lewis R & Rourke D. Differentiation of temporal lobe and generalized seizure patients with the WAIS. *J Consult Clin Psychol*, 1980, 48:39-42.

Milner B. Psychological deficits produced by temporal lobe excision. *Res Pub Assoc Res Nerv Mental Dis*, 1958, 36:244-257.

Milner B. Visual recognition and recall after right temporal excision in man. *Neuropsychologia*, 1968, 6:191-209.

Milner B. Disorders of learning and memory after temporal lobe lesions in man. *Clin Neurosurg*, 1972, 19:421-446.

Milner B. (1975). Psychological aspects of focal epilepsy and its neurosurgical management. In: DP Purpura, JK Penry, & RD Walter (eds.), *Advances in neurology* (pp. 299-321). New York: Raven Press.

Milner B. (1986). Memory and the human brain. In: M Shafto (ed.), *How we know* (pp. 31-59). San Francisco: Harper & Row.

Mirsky AF. (1989). Information processing in petit mal epilepsy. In BP Hermann & M Seidenberg (eds.), *Childhood epilepsies: Neuropsychological, psychosocial and intervention aspects* (pp. 51–70). Chichester: John Wiley & Sons.

Mirsky AF & Van Buren JM. On the nature of the "absence" in centrencephalic epilepsy: A study of some behavioral, electroencephalographic and autonomic factors. *Electroenceph Clin Neurophysiol*, 1965, 18:334–348.

Moehele KA, Bolter JF & Long CJ. The relationship between neuropsychological functioning and psychopathology in temporal lobe epileptic patients. *Epilepsia*, 1984, 25:418–422.

Moses JA, Csernansky JG & Leiderman DB. Neuropsychological criteria for identification of cognitive deficits in limbic epilepsy. *Int J Clin Neuropsychol*, 1988, 10:106–112.

Mungas D, Ehlers C, Walton N & McCutchen CB. Verbal learning differences in epileptic patients with left and right temporal lobe foci. *Epilepsia*, 1985, 26:340–345.

Novelly RA, Augustine EA, Mattson RH, Glaser G, Williamson PD, Spencer DD & Spencer SS. Selective memory improvement and impairment in temporal lobectomy for epilepsy. *Ann Neurol*, 1984, 15:64–67.

O'Leary D, Seidenberg M, Berent S & Boll TJ. The effects of age of onset of tonic-clonic seizures on neuropsychological performance of children. *Epilepsia*, 1981, 22:197–203.

O'Leary D, Lovell MR, Sackellares JC, Berent S, Giordani B, Seidenberg M & Boll TJ. Effects of age of onset of partial and generalized seizures on neuropsychological performance in children. *J Nerv Ment Dis*, 1983, 171:624–629.

Parsons OA & Kemp DE. Intellectual functioning in temporal lobe epilepsy. *J Consult Clin Psychol*, 1960, 24:408–414.

Paskind HA. Extramural patients with epilepsy with special reference to the frequent absence of deterioration. *Arch Neurol Psychiatry*, 1932, 28:370–385.

Paskind HA. The absence of deteriorating effects of bromides in epilepsy. *J Am Med Assoc*, 1934, 103:100–103.

Patterson HA & Fonner D. Some observations on the intelligence quotient in epileptics. *Psychiatric Quarterly*, 1928, 12:542–548.

Pazzaglia P & Frank-Pazzaglia L. Record in grade school of pupils with epilepsy: An epidemiological study. *Epilepsia*, 1976, 17:361–366.

Pihl RO. The degree of the verbal-performance discrepancy on the WISC and the WAIS and severity of EEG abnormality in epileptics. *J Clin Psychol*, 1968, 24:418–420.

Rausch R & Babb TL. (1987). Evidence for memory specialization within the mesial temporal lobe in man. In: J Engel, GA Ojemann, HO Luders & PD Williamson (eds.), *Fundamental mechanisms of human brain function* (pp. 103–109). New York: Raven Press.

Rausch R, Lieb JP & Crandall P. Neuropsychologic correlates of depth spike activity in epileptic patients. *Arch Neurol*, 1978, 35:699–705.

Rutter M, Graham P & Yule WA. (1970). *A neuropsychiatric study in childhood*. London: SIMP Heinemann Medical.

Sackellares JC, Giordani B, Berent S, Seidenberg M, Dreifuss FE, Vanderzant CW & Boll TJ. Patients with pseudoseizures: Intellectual and cognitive performance. *Neurology*, 1985, 35:116-119.

Sass KJ, Spencer DD, Kim JH, Westerveld M, Novelly RA & Lencz T. Verbal memory impairment correlates with hippocampal pyramidal cell density. *Neurology*, 1990, 40:1694-1697.

Schain RJ, Ward JW & Guthrie D. Carbamazepine as an anticonvulsant in children. *Neurology*, 1977, 27:476-480.

Schwab RS. A method of measuring consciousness in petit mal epilepsy. *J Nerv Ment Dis*, 1939, 89:690-691.

Schwartz ML, Dennerll RD & Lin Y. Neuropsychological and psychosocial predictors of employability in epilepsy. *J Clin Psychol*, 1968, 24:174-177.

Seidenberg M. (1989a). Academic achievement and school performance of children with epilepsy. In: BP Hermann & M Seidenberg (eds.), *Childhood epilepsies: Neuropsychological, psychosocial and intervention aspects* (pp. 105-118). Chichester: John Wiley & Sons.

Seidenberg M. (1989b). Neuropsychological functioning of children with epilepsy. In: BP Hermann & M Seidenberg (eds.), *Childhood epilepsies: Neuropsychological, psychosocial and intervention aspects* (pp. 71-81). Chichester: John Wiley & Sons.

Seidenberg M, Beck N, Geisser M, Giordani B, Sackellares JC, Berent S, Dreifuss FE & Boll TJ. Academic achievement of children with epilepsy. *Epilepsia*, 1986, 27:753-759.

Seidenberg M, Beck N, Geisser M, O'Leary D, Giordani B, Berent S, Sackellares JC, Dreifuss FE & Boll TJ. Neuropsychological correlates of academic achievement of children with epilepsy. *J Epilepsy*, 1987, 1:23-30.

Seidenberg, M, O'Leary, DS, Berent, S & Boll, T. Changes in seizure frequency and test-retest scores on the Wechsler Adult Intelligence Scale. *Epilepsia*, 1981a, 22:75-83.

Seidenberg M, O'Leary DS, Giordani B, Berent S & Boll TJ. Test-retest IQ changes of epilepsy patients: Assessing the influence of practice effects. *J Clin Neuropsychol*, 1981b, 3:237-255.

Shalman DC. The diagnostic use of the McGill Picture Anomaly test in temporal lobe epilepsy. *J Neurol Neurosurg Psychiatry*, 1961, 24:220-222.

Shewmon DA & Erwin RJ. The effect of focal interictal spikes on perception and reaction time: I. General considerations. *EEG Clin Neurophysiol*, 1988a, 69: 319-337.

Shewmon DA & Erwin RJ. The effect of focal interictal spikes on perception and reaction time. II. Neuroanatomic specificity. *EEG Clin Neurophysiol*, 1988b, 69:338-352.

Shewmon DA & Erwin RJ. Focal spike-induced cerebral dysfunction is related to the after-coming slow wave. *Ann Neurol*, 1988c, 23:131-137.

Simmel ML & Counts S. (1958). Clinical and psychological results of anterior temporal lobectomy in patients with psychomotor epilepsy. In: M Baldwin & P Bailey (eds.), *Temporal lobe epilepsy* (pp. 1247-1261). Springfield: Charles C. Thomas.

Somerfeld-Ziskind E & Ziskind E. Effect of phenobarbital on the mentality of epileptic patients. *Arch Neurol Psychiatry*, 1940, 43:70-79.

Stafiniak P, Saykin AJ, Sperling MR, Kester MS, Robinson LJ, O'Connor MJ & Gur RC. Acute naming deficits following dominant anterior temporal lobectomy: Prediction by age at first risk for seizures. *Neurology*, 1990, 40:1509-1512.

Stevens JR. (1975). Interictal clinical manifestations of complex partial seizures. In: JK Penry & DD Daly (eds.), *Advances in neurology* (pp. 85-112). New York: Raven Press.

Stores G. Reading skills of children with generalized or focal epilepsy attending ordinary school. *Dev Med Child Neurol*, 1976, 18:705-716.

Taylor LB. (1979). Psychological assessment of neurosurgical patients. In: T Rasmussen (ed.), *Functional neurosurgery* (pp. 163-180). New York: Raven Press.

Tarter RE. Intellectual and adaptive functioning in epilepsy: A review of 50 years of research. *Dis Nerv Sys*, 1972, 33:763-770.

Thompson PJ. (1983). Phenytoin and psychosocial development. In: PL Morselli, CE Pippenger & JK Penry (eds.), *Antiepileptic drug therapy in pediatrics* (pp. 159-167). New York: Raven Press.

Tizard B & Margerison JH. Psychological functions during spike-wave discharge. *Br J Soc Clin Psychol*, 1963, 3:6-15.

Trimble MR. Dementia in epilepsy. *Acta Neurol Scand*, 1984, 69(Suppl. 99):99-104.

Trimble MR & Thompson PJ. Sodium valproate and cognitive function. *Epilepsia*, 1984, 25(Suppl. 99):S60-S64.

Trostle JA, Hauser WA & Sharbrough FW. Psychological and social adjustment to epilepsy in Rochester, Minnesota. *Neurology*, 1989, 39:633-637.

Tucker DM, Novelly RA, Isaac W & Spencer D. Effects of simultaneous vs sequential stimulus presentation of memory performance following temporal lobe resection in humans. *Neuropsychologia*, 1986, 24:277-281.

Wannamaker BB & Matthews CG. Prognostic implications of neuropsychologic test performance for surgical treatment of epilepsy. *J Nerv Ment Dis*, 1976, 163:29-34.

Wapner I, Thurston DL & Holowach J. Phenobarbital: Its effect on learning in epileptic children. *J Am Med Assoc*, 1962, 182:139.

Wilkus RJ & Dodrill C. Neuropsychological correlates of the electroencephalogram in epileptics: I. Topographic distribution and average rate of epileptiform discharges. *Epilepsia*, 1976, 17:89-100.

Wilkus RJ, Dodrill C & Thompson PM. Intensive EEG monitoring and psychological studies of patients with pseudoepileptic seizures. *Epilepsia*, 1984, 25:100-107.

Yacorzynski GK & Arieff AJ. Absence of deterioration in patients with non-organic epilepsy with special reference to bromide therapy. *J Nerv Ment Dis*, 1942, 95:687-697.

Zielinski JJ. (1986). Selected psychiatric and psychosocial aspects of epilepsy as seen by an epidemiologist. In: S Whitman & BP Hermann (eds.), *Psychopathology in epilepsy: Social dimensions* (pp. 36-65). New York: Oxford University Press.

2

When Is Computer-Assisted Testing Appropriate?

Carl B. Dodrill

Regional Epilepsy Center
University of Washington School of Medicine, Seattle, Washington

Introduction

A great deal of information has been presented at this conference which bears on the topic of the appropriateness of computer-assisted testing. Despite this fact, however, the answer to the question of when it is appropriate is not necessarily straightforward. At the minimum, the correct response is likely to vary from one investigation to the next depending on the particular medication under study, the type of investigation, the amount of money available to undertake it, how many testing sites will be involved, the technical expertise available to support the project, and so forth. In view of these factors and others, it is unrealistic to expect that a single and universal answer will ultimately be found.

An important fact which is apparent from the literature on the cognitive effects of antiepileptic drugs is that in any given investigation, there is a strong tendency to either use computer-assisted procedures entirely or not to use them at all. While occasional exceptions are found (Aldenkamp et al. 1987; Thompson et al. 1981), literature is lacking which would help provide guidelines as to when computer-assisted testing might be more appropriate than using standardized neuropsychological tests, when the reverse might be true, or when both are equally appropriate. Clearly this places us at a disadvantage in our efforts to obtain the answer to the basic question at hand.

As an investigator who has now used computer-assisted procedures for several years *in combination with* standardized neuropsychological tests, I have become convinced that at least four conditions must be met in order for computer-assisted testing to be appropriate. These conditions are detailed below along with literature citations insofar as they exist.

Conditions Required for Computer-Assisted Testing

The conditions for this testing (discussed here) are considered to be a minimum; there is no intention to create an exhaustive list. It will be noted that the conditions mentioned here vary somewhat from those presented elsewhere in this volume. This is to be expected in an area that is relatively new because quite different approaches have evolved at various locations around the world.

1. Availability of Technical Expertise for Hardware Construction and Maintenance

The degree of difficulty incurred in meeting this condition is dependent on the type of hardware utilized. There are two basic types of hardware systems used with this type of testing in the world today. The first of these is a self-contained computer system. In this system, a standard computer is used, typically with a standard keyboard. A standard monitor may also be employed although custom monitors are sometimes utilized including those with a touch screen. Regardless of the exact details of the system, the hallmark of the system is that it utilizes equipment, which is commercially available, and typically no other hardware.

The second type of system is one in which a computer drives and records information from *peripheral* equipment to which the subject both attends and responds. A standard monitor and keyboard are also included in this system, but they are available only to the person administering the test. In the most commonly used configuration of this type, the computer is programmed to drive a slide projector that delivers stimuli at predetermined times and for the precise intervals specified by the software (Aman et al. 1987; Dodrill 1991; Thompson et al. 1981). The patient usually registers responses with the aid of a response box that may consist of as few as two response buttons ("Yes" and "No").

An example of this second type of system is the system I use in my own research. An IBM-compatible 286 microprocessor computer is adjacent to the slide projector. The computer operates the slide projector by means of a specially constructed board inside the computer box. This board has its own clock so that it does not depend on the clock built in the computer to keep time. The board also operates a tachistoscopic shutter placed on the slide projector. The entire apparatus is enclosed in two ventilated soundproof boxes that reduce noise and keep the equipment from raising the room temperature. The operator utilizes a standard keyboard and monitor in order to activate the software.

Images from the slide projector are projected on a screen 6 feet away from the subject and at eye level. The computer screen is not seen by the subject who operates a two-button response pad ("Yes" and "No").

Advantages and disadvantages with each of the above systems are evident. The self-contained computer systems are far easier to construct and at least somewhat easier to maintain. This is an especially important point if one anticipates a study that would utilize multiple testing sites. Portability is also clearly better. One disadvantage of the self-contained system is that it utilizes a standard computer keyboard with which some subjects are far more familiar (and less intimidated by) than others. A second disadvantage is the fact that unless one modifies the computer internally, one is limited in accuracy to 17 msec (1/60th of a second) because screen updates occur at this rate. In those countries where 50 Hz current is utilized, screen updates occur every 20 msec. It is unclear whether this degree of error is important in studies of the cognitive effects of antiepileptic drugs, but note that often a 50 msec difference between two drug conditions will result in a statistically significant difference (Aman et al. 1990).

The advantages and disadvantages of the second type of computer system are largely complimentary with the first. A good tachistoscopic shutter can open with no more than a 10-msec delay and by hyperpowering the impulse which opens (but not which sustains the opening of) the shutter, one can reduce the latency to approximately 5 msec. Thus the error with this system is minimal. Another advantage of this system is that extremely complex stimuli, such as complex color photographs, can be presented with minimal delay and without the requiring of sizable computer memory for storage. This is difficult with a self-contained computer system because a color palette of at least 256 (and preferably 512) colors is needed to form a picture of excellent quality. Such a palette would require a huge capacity for memory storage. The final significant advantage is that the response equipment can be tailor-made to suit various purposes and populations (Aman et al. 1987) so that it is widely adaptable. In my own work, for example, it has been possible to construct an automobile braking simulator that can be hooked up to the computer instead of the hand-operated response pad. Disadvantages include greater difficulty in original construction, diminished portability, and less adaptability to a multisite operation. In my experience, the original construction of the system posed the greatest difficulty.

Overall, the choice of hardware systems depends on the needs of the proposed study, the required number of study sites, and the necessary accuracy in measurement. Whether computed-assisted procedures can be used at all will of course depend on the availability of several thousand dollars for each testing unit. Finally, there must be at least some capability for hardware repair and maintenance. Thus hardware considerations represent an area of significant initial importance in identifying circumstances when computerized testing is appropriate.

2. Technical Expertise Must Be Available
to Construct and Maintain the Necessary Software

This second requirement for computer-assisted testing is time consuming and requires significant expertise. Every facility utilizing computer-assisted testing known to me has been forced to employ at least one computer programmer initially and also to have someone at hand who can resolve problems in the programs as they arise. Occasionally, problems appear in these programs only months after they have been in use, and even though some of these problems are small, they demand attention. Rather than any form of Basic, a high-level language such as Pascal or C is very desirable in order to facilitate the construction of complex programmatic designs and to promote the rapid execution of commands. Adequate documentation within the programs is highly desirable in order to permit further modifications and refinements at a much later date when the original programmer is unavailable. Finally, subject response must be backed up (stored) frequently in order to prevent the loss of data in the event of computer failure.

Eventually, it should be possible to utilize in many epilepsy centers software that was constructed at a single center. At the present time, however, there has been very little use of such an approach both because the hardware differences across the centers are substantial and also because there has not always been adequate communication between the centers. For example, the programs used in the early work by Thompson et al. (1981) in the United Kingdom were kindly made available to me, but no computer system could be found in the United States which could read them. All programs had to then be redone, and changes were inevitably introduced.

The design of the tests to be administered constitutes a significant challenge. In this text, Kinsbourne presents a set of testing procedures well based in cognitive theory and which merit further consideration. It is yet to be determined whether such procedures are more sensitive to antiepileptic drugs than the clinically based systems that are utilized in most centers, but efforts should certainly be made to test them.

3. Computer-Assisted Tests Must Bring Promise of
Greater Sensitivity to Drug Effects

There is little reason to undertake the expense and substantial amount of work required to set up a computer-assisted system if there is not at least some hope that such a system will (a) tap areas not normally covered by standard neuropsychological tests, or (b) improve accuracy and precision in measurement. Reasons why computer-assisted tests might perform well in this context are not difficult to find, however. First, it is certainly possible to present stimuli with greater precision and to record responses more accurately with computer-assisted tests than with standard neuropsychological tests. Also, many people are more interested in material presented by computers, and this may help to maintain fuller cooperation, possibly for a longer period of time. Additionally, it would appear that certain types of mental processes could be better tested with a computer-assisted approach than with standard neuropsychological tests. Reference is made to Kinsbourne's chapter in the present volume for a further discussion of these issues.

Whereas there are certainly reasons why computer-assisted tests *might* be more sensitive to drug effects than standard neuropsychological tests, the question remains as to whether this is in fact the case. As was indicated earlier in this chapter, there is a strong tendency for investigators to utilize computer-assisted tests or standard neuropsychological tests in a given study, but not both. Where both types of tests have been reported, there has been no deliberate effort to compare the two approaches in terms of sensitivity to drug effects. Thus, there is a dearth of evidence that clearly shows computer-assisted procedures to be sufficiently superior to justify the amount of time and money required by the approach. To help shed light on this important area, some time ago I began to collect data on both systems of assessment with the same group of patients, and preliminary results are reported below.

The purpose of the study was to determine to what degree computer-assisted tests would reflect major changes in antiepileptic drug serum levels in comparison with standard neuropsychological tests. Fifteen surgical candidates (9 men, 6 women) with partial seizures, averaging 31.87 years of age (SD = 10.08) and 12.64 years of education (SD = 1.78), were hospitalized for long-term EEG monitoring in an effort to record several typical seizures. To promote the appearance of seizures, all of these patients had one and only one major drug reduced or completely stopped. All subjects were tested twice with a low-

TABLE 1

Dose and Serum Level Data on the Drug which was Changed

			Low Serum Level		High Serum Level	
Drug	N		M	SD	M	SD
Carbamazepine	8	Dose	294	423	1,112	336
		SL	2.5	2.4	8.4	1.0
Valproate	3	Dose	0.0	0.0	1,313	577
		SL	0.0	0.0	43.3	18.2
Phenytoin	2	Dose	200	212	400	0.0
		SL	8.7	12.0	25.6	19.6
Phenobarbital	2	Dose	0.0	0.0	295	290
		SL	0.0	0.0	17.5	6.2

Notes: M = mean, SD = standard deviation, SL = serum level.

TABLE 2

Mean Scores on All Test Measures

Test/Variable	Low Drug		High Drug		Significance
	Mean	SD	Mean	SD	
Standard Neuropsychological Tests					
Name writing (let/sec)	1.03	.33	.98	.30	NS
Wonderlic Personnel Test, IQ	90.00	16.28	93.00	15.23	NS
Wonderlic Personnel Test, errors	8.75	8.27	7.50	6.02	NS
Digit Symbol Modalities	45.42	12.71	43.08	11.23	NS
Stroop, reading speed (sec)	51.40	24.98	47.53	14.11	NS
Stroop, interference (sec)	138.87	120.17	166.53	237.79	NS
Digit Cancellation, correct	124.82	28.33	119.09	41.60	NS
Digit Cancellation, omits	1.45	2.21	3.81	2.93	$p < .05$
Finger Tapping, preferred hand	51.17	6.77	50.00	6.10	NS
Auditory Verbal Learning	23.71	5.89	24.14	8.11	NS
Computer-Assisted Tests					
Simple Reaction Time					
5 trial short delay (msec)	313.29	174.00	309.71	161.90	NS
10 trial short delay (msec)	229.93	60.57	249.29	111.72	NS
10 trial long delay (msec)	223.43	38.82	276.07	79.61	$p < .03$
Choice Reaction Time					
Latency (msec)	699.82	234.71	745.41	262.47	NS
Number items correct	57.00	2.96	56.14	3.84	NS
Name Learning					
Latency (msec)	3,335.71	919.12	4,042.57	913.55	$p < .003$
Number items correct	20.29	7.40	16.50	7.76	$p < .02$
Unanswered items	5.57	5.37	6.43	4.55	NS
Decision Making					
Latency (msec)	757.40	255.00	802.13	364.76	NS
Number items correct	55.87	4.26	56.40	2.97	NS

Note: NS = not significant.

versus high-drug order counterbalanced (in 8 cases, the first testing was with reduced medication and in 7 it was the second testing that had the reduced medication). Average doses and drug serum levels on the drug which was changed are presented in Table 1 for both the low and the high conditions. As can be seen, the differences between the low and high serum levels were very substantial. The drug which was reduced was most commonly carbamazepine.

The results of the study are presented in Table 2, first for the standard neuropsychological tests and then for the computer-assisted procedures. Speed of writing one's name has been associated with antiepileptic serum levels (Dodrill 1975), as have scores on a brief measure of intelligence, the Wonderlic Personnel Test (Dodrill & Troupin 1977). The Stroop Test arises from the Neuropsychological Battery for Epilepsy (Dodrill 1978) and consists of a simple reading condition (Part I) as well as the more difficult interference condition (Part II). The first half of the original test was used but with alternate forms on the two testings. On the Digit Cancellation Test, two digits were canceled in a page of single-digit numbers over the course of a 3-minute period. Both the number of items correct and the number of omitted items were counted. The Finger Tapping Test is from the Halstead-Reitan Neuropsychological Battery for Adults and is part of the Neuropsychological Battery for Epilepsy. Finally, the Three Trial Auditory Verbal Learning Test consisted of alternate forms of 15-item word lists that are controlled for frequency of word usage according to the Thorndike-Lorge word lists (Thorndike & Lorge 1944). This test is patterned after the Rey Auditory Verbal Learning Test (Rey 1964), and the score rendered is the total number of correct items for the three trials.

Out of all these test variables, only the number of items omitted on the Digit Cancellation Test produced a statistically significant difference. While this difference was in the expected direction, it certainly represents a minimal finding considering the significant changes in drug levels that were made.

Turning to the computer-assisted measures, Simple Reaction Time was patterned in part after that of Thompson et al. (1981). The light appears from the slide projector on the screen without the illumination of a slide, and the patient hits the response button as quickly as possible. Both for the initial 5 warm-up trials and for the next 10 trials, short intervals of 0.5–2 s were used, which randomly varied in length between the last response and the appearance of the next stimulus. These trials were followed by 10 long interval trials, which varied between 1 and 10 s between presentation of the stimuli. The measures obtained were the average latencies for each group of trials.

The measure of choice reaction time was the People Test, which consists of a series of 60 photographs in which people are either conspicuously present or else they are not present at all. The subjects hit the "Yes" button if people are present and the "No" button if they are not present. Latency in milliseconds (msec) as well as the number of items correct are recorded.

The Name Learning Test consists of the presentation of a series of 12 pictures of young men and women along with an orally given first name for each. After each has been exposed for 10-s periods, a recall trial follows with presentation of each picture again in random order with recall of the names requested. Up to 10 s per response is allowed for each item. This entire procedure is completed a total of three times and the total number of correct and unanswered items are recorded as well as the mean latency for all 36 trials.

The final computer-assisted test, which we use, is the Decision Making Test. This test is only slightly modified from Thompson et al. (1981). A total of 60 items are included consisting of red or black line drawings of animate or inanimate objects. Before the appearance of each, the examiner asks, "Is it red?" or "Is it alive?" Both the number of items correct and the mean latency are recorded.

Results from all these computer-assisted procedures are presented in Table 2. There are three statistically significant differences, all of which are in the expected direction. Therefore, the results of this study provide at least some evidence to suggest that computer-assisted tests may have a place in the assessment of the cognitive effects of antiepileptic drugs, and that they may provide information not obtained by standard neuropsychological tests. Even a measure of simple reaction time may be of some assistance if an effort is made to vary the length of the intervals between the trials and in particular to include trials with longer intertrial intervals. The results of the Name Learning Test are of significant interest not only because more items were correct with lower serum drug levels but also because the latency for response in this more complex memory task achieved a difference of 700 msec between the low and high drug level conditions. This is a remarkably great difference when compared with results of other studies of antiepileptic drugs. It could represent a degree of slowing that is significant with respect to performance in everyday life. Such a small difference could never be detected using a stopwatch with standard neuropsychological procedures, however.

The results of this preliminary study must obviously be interpreted with caution. Clearly, a far larger number of subjects is needed with an adequate sample for each drug which is reduced. Until then, one can only hope that other investigators will also compare computer-assisted tests with standard neuropsychological procedures so that ultimately more definitive statements can be made about the drug sensitivity of these two methods.

4. Computer-Assisted Tests Must Have the Probability of Finding a Meaningful Difference

The question has been justifiably raised as to whether or not some of the statistically significant differences noted from computer-assisted tests have any practical significance, and if so, what such differences mean. A statistically significant result does not necessarily represent a worthwhile difference. For example, studies have frequently reported that white blood cell counts diminish significantly with the addition of carbamazepine to a drug regimen, but this finding is truly meaningless unless such counts diminish to a clinically significant level. Of what practical significance is the result presented in Table 2 that a 50-msec difference exists with respect to simple reaction time with long intertrial intervals? Could such a delay have an impact on driving an automobile, for example? If in fact a person is 50 msec slower in getting to the brake pedal while driving at 55 mph, only 4 more feet would be required to stop the vehicle (232 feet instead of 228 feet) in an emergency situation. Is this a difference of practical significance? It is in fact difficult to think of occupations in which a small difference in latency would have any clear effect. It may of course be that the simple model proposed here is inadequate and that there are several cognitive processes that must occur, each of which would perhaps be delayed by 50 msec. Clearly more information is required concerning the practical significance of test findings.

The second question dealing with the meaning of the results pertains to the type of functions measured by the various tests. In this area, it has been easy for investigators to look at a test and on the basis of its apparent content to make a decision about what they believe the test measures. After this decision has been made, there is little questioning as to whether or not a correct conclusion has been reached. For example, one might ask: What does the Decision Making Test actually measure? Is the primary cognitive activity it evaluates truly "ability to make decisions" or problem-solving ability?

The importance of the question at hand can be illustrated with data from 47 adults with epilepsy who received the computer-assisted tests described above plus the complete Neuropsychological Battery for Epilepsy. The tests were

TABLE 3

Correlation of Decision Making Latency with Other Tests
(N = 47)

Problem Solving		Motor Speed	
Category Test	.60**	Finger Tapping	-.62**
TPT, Time	.48**	Name Writing	-.62**
Trail Making B	.58**	Marching Test, Time	.69**
Attention/Concentration		Intelligence	
Digit Span	.60**	WAIS-R Verbal IQ	-.42*
Stroop, interference	.73**	WAIS-R Performance IQ	-.50**
Tonal Memory	-.37*	WAIS-R Full Scale IQ	-.49**

Notes: *$p < .01$. **$p < .001$.

divided according to four basic constructs with only those procedures included here, which have a very major loading on one of these. The average latency on the Decision Making Test was then correlated (Pearson r) with the test measures within each of the four groups, and the results are presented in Table 3. An examination of the data from this table reveals that Decision Making is correlated to a substantial degree with variables in each of the four areas, so that it defies clear-cut classification. It is perhaps discouraging to note that this test correlates most consistently with measures of motor speed, a construct which, to my knowledge, no one has ever claimed it measures. Nevertheless, one can see this as a possibility because the time required to get to the response button is obviously very important. Attention/Concentration and Problem Solving appear to be about equally related to Decision Making, and Intelligence is somewhat less related. While the data presented on Table 3 do not present the final answers concerning what this particularly well-known test evaluates, they do draw our attention to the important question of what these tests actually measure.

Conclusions

As was indicated at the beginning of this chapter, the answer to the question "When is a computer-assisted testing appropriate?" is complex, and it is almost certain that there is no one answer for all situations. For any given particular study, however, the following general guidelines are recommended for consideration:

1. There must be sufficient funds and technical expertise to construct and maintain the hardware. The type of hardware selected should depend on the requirements of the study and should be considered in connection with the advantages and disadvantages of the two basic types of hardware detailed above.

2. There must be sufficient expertise to construct and service the software. Debugging the software is essential. It is desirable to include theoretical considerations in test selection.

3. It is highly desirable to include both computer-assisted and standard neuropsychological tests in any study. This will provide for a broader range of assessment of functions and also for a comparison of the sensitivity of the two general types of measures.

4. The tests should be interpreted with caution both in terms of the practical significance of the findings and also with respect to what the particular procedures are believed to measure.

Careful consideration of each of these factors will lead to a more rational selection of tests in this area. This should provide assistance for the more appropriate selection of both standard neuropsychological and computer-assisted measures in studies of antiepileptic drug effects.

Acknowledgments

A portion of the research reported in this chapter was supported in NIH grants NS 17111 and NS 24823 awarded by the National Institute of Neurological Disorders and Stroke, PHS/DHHS. Linda M. Ojemann, M.D. and Alan J. Wilensky, M.D. provided the subjects used in the studies reported in this chapter.

References

Aldenkamp AP, Alpherts WCJ, Moerland MC, Ottevanger N & Van Parys JAP. Controlled release carbamazepine: Cognitive side effects in patients with epilepsy. *Epilepsia*, 1987, 28:507-514.

Aman MG, Werry, JS, Paxton JW & Turbott SH. Effect of sodium valproate on psychomotor performance in children as a function of dose, fluctuations in concentration, and diagnosis. *Epilepsia*, 1987, 28:115-114.

Aman MG, Werry JS, Paxton JW, Turbott, SH & Stewart AW. Effects of carbamazepine on psychomotor performance in children as a function of drug concentration, seizure type, and time of medication. *Epilepsia*, 1990, 31:51-60.

Dodrill CB. Diphenylhydantoin serum levels, toxicity, and neuropsychological performance in patients with epilepsy. *Epilepsia*, 1975, 16:593-600.

Dodrill CB. A neuropsychological battery for epilepsy. *Epilepsia*, 1978, 19:611-623.

Dodrill CB. (1991). Behavioral effects of antiepileptic drugs. In: D Smith & MR Trimble (eds.), *Neurobehavioral problems in epilepsy: Advances in neurology* (vol. 55) (pp. 213-224). New York: Raven Press.

Dodrill CB & Troupin AS. Psychotropic effects of carbamazepine in epilepsy: A double-blind comparison with phenytoin. *Neurology*, 1977, 27:1023-1028.

Rey A. (1964). *L'examen clinique en psychologie*. Paris: Presses Universitaries de France.

Thompson PJ, Huppert FA & Trimble MR. Phenytoin and cognitive function: Effects on normal volunteers. *Br J Soc Clin Psychol*, 1981, 20:155-162.

Thorndike EL & Lorge I. (1944). *The teacher's word book of 30,000 words*. New York: Columbia University Press.

———— **3** ————

Integrating Computerized and Traditional Neuropsychological Assessment Techniques

Pamela J. Thompson

Epilepsy Research Group, National Hospitals, Chalfont Centre for Epilepsy
London, England

We are shortly moving into the phase where computers will become one of the cheapest pieces of technology on Earth—cheaper than TV sets, cheaper even than transistor radios. They will for exactly the same reasons become the most common pieces of technology in the world and the most useful (Evans 1979).

Introduction

Computer applications, as Evans (1979) predicted, are being made in almost every area of human endeavor and neuropsychological assessment is no exception. Despite the increase in availability of computerized techniques, these are often given limited coverage in neuropsychological texts that cover assessment techniques. Thus it is timely to consider the role of computerized assessment in the neuropsychological evaluation of epilepsy.

Computerized neuropsychological assessment can have a role in the administration, scoring, analysis, interpretation of results, and in report writing. In addition, vast quantities of data pertaining to many dimensions of a subject's test performance can be stored economically.

Test Interpretation

Computer-based scoring and interpretation of psychological tests—including neuropsychological measures—have the longest history, although it appears to be more prevalent in the United States than in Europe (Fowler 1985). Four neuropsychological interpretational programs reflecting differing conceptual schemes are outlined by Adams and Heaton (1985) in their review of the area.

Several interpretational programs are commercially available. Table 1 lists interpretational programs taken from the *Psychware Sourcebook* (Krug 1988). There are programs that provide interpretations for specific tests such as the Wechsler Scale and the Halstead–Reitan Battery, and also measures like the Report Writer Adult Intellectual Achievement and Neuropsychological Screen that take into account scores on a variety of measures. The developers explain "this program provides integrated interpretations of the WAIS-R, Stanford–Binet, WRAT, WRAT-R, Stroop Color Word Test, Trail Making Test, Aphasia Screening, Signs and Symbol Digit Modalities Test." Adams and Heaton (1985) acknowledge that there is a wide margin for improvement in the automated interpretation of neuropsychological test data programs. However, they write

TABLE 1

Commercially Available Computerized Neuropsychological Test Interpretation Programs

Halstead–Reitan Hypothesis Generator	Report Writer; WAIS-R
Halstead–Reitan Neuropsychology Battery	Report Writer; WISC-R
Halstead–Reitan Interpretation for Adults	WAIS-R Analysis II
Halstead–Reitan Interpretation for Older Adults	WAIS-R Microcomputer-Assisted Interpretative Report
IQ Test Interpretation—Adult (WAIS-R)	WAIS-R Narrative Report
IQ Test Interpretation—Clinical (WAIS-R)	WAIS-R Report Version 3.0
IQ Test Interpretation—Educational (WISC-R)	WAIS-Riter Basic
Luria Nebraska Neuropsychological Battery	WAIS-Riter Complete
Luria Nebraska Scoring System	Weathers WISC-R/WAIS-R Reports
Report Writer; Adults' Intellectual Achievement and Neuropsychological Screening	Wechsler Interpretation System
Report Writer; Children's Intellectual and Achievement Tests	WISC-R Analysis II

(The table continues with the following entries in the right column: WAIS-R Analysis II, WAIS-R Microcomputer-Assisted Interpretative Report, WAIS-R Narrative Report, WAIS-R Report Version 3.0, WAIS-Riter Basic, WAIS-Riter Complete, Weathers WISC-R/WAIS-R Reports, Wechsler Interpretation System, WISC-R Analysis II, WISC-R Compilation: Software Adaptation, WISC-R Microcomputer-Assisted Interpretative Report, WISC-R Report Version 3.0, WISC-R Riter Basic, WISC-R Riter Complete, WIPPSI Analysis II, WIPPSI Report Version II)

Note: From Krug (1988).

that given a specific range of diagnostic alternatives in data sources the diagnostic accuracy of a well designed computerized decision program should exceed that of the clinical neuropsychologist in combining the same data.

Test Administration

Accounts of computerized neuropsychological administration consider the system described by Elwood and Griffin (1972) as a landmark (Fowler 1985). This was not computer based but used a variety of machines to simulate the traditional administration of the WAIS. Gilberstadt and colleagues (1976) described an automated system of intelligence test delivery and report writing. The tests administered included the Shipley–Hartford Vocabulary Test, the Raven's Progressive Matrices, the WAIS Digit Span and Halstead Category Test. Stimuli were projected on the console screen by a slide projection mechanism. Responses were given by depressing keys on the console. Reaction time was measured and automatically recorded. The system also generated computerized reports.

It was the arrival of the microcomputer that resulted in an increase in the development of automated testing systems. Today, many neuropsychological tests are available for use on a personal computer. Here, three systems developed in the United Kingdom will be briefly mentioned.

One of the earliest pioneers of microcomputer neuropsychological test administration was Elithorn. Together with colleagues he has developed a series of computerized psychological tests; probably the best known is the Perceptual Maze Test (Elithorn et al. 1982). This is a tracking measure, which requires the subject to find a path through a lattice of dots, to pass either through the maximum number of dots possible or a specified number of dots. The task difficulty can be varied according to the size of the lattice. Other tests in the battery include a digit-span memory test, a coding test, a tracking test, a memory test for nonsense syllables and words, a tapping test, a reaction time test, a reading speed and vigilance task, and a vocabulary test. Elithorn and coworkers report that these tests are useful in assessing patients, particularly in monitoring the effects of intervention. Studied to date have been the effects of levodopa therapy on patients with chronic hepatic encephalopathy (Elithorn et al. 1975) and drug treatment in psychiatric patients (Elithorn et al. 1982).

Acker (1983) reports a microcomputer-based neuropsychological assessment system that was standardized during work with detoxified alcoholics. Acker's aim was to develop a battery of new tests which would fully exploit the strengths of the microcomputer. The tests were written for the Commodore PET series of microcomputers and used in conjunction with a specially designed keyboard, such that subjects were presented with only those alternative responses that were appropriate for a particular test. The tests were designed to assess visuospatial ability, perceptual motor speed, visual perceptual analysis, verbal recognition memory, visuospatial memory, and abstract thinking. Results obtained with each of the tests were correlated with those obtained on the standard psychometric version similar to the automated test. For each such comparison the correlation coefficients were significant but low.

Beaumont and French (1987) described a microcomputer-aided cognitive battery, which includes versions of neuropsychological measures designed to be as similar as possible to the standard version. These were the Mill Hill Vocabulary Test, the Differential Aptitude Test of Language Use and Spelling, Raven's Progressive Matrices, the Wisconsin Card Sorting Test, the Digit Span Test, and the Money Road Map Test. The authors assessed the usefulness and validity of the computer-generated measures in a large survey. Three hundred and sixty-seven patients were randomly allocated to standard or automated testing, and, if automated, to keyboard or touch screen peripherals. Patients were retested using the alternative form within 33 to 60 days. Reliability coefficients between automated (computerized) and standard formats were significant but varied. The highest correlations occurred with the Mill Hill Vocabulary Test, which led the authors to conclude that the automated and standard version of this measure were psychometrically equivalent. For the other tests the reliability coefficients were not sufficiently high enough for the authors to conclude such equivalence. Beaumont and French (1987) rightly point out that although the computerized tests were not the same as the traditional measure this does not mean that they have no clinical value.

Today, a variety of computerized neuropsychological tests are commercially available and it is likely that there are many more idiosyncratic systems being

TABLE 2

A Sample of Commercially Available Computerized Neuropsychological Test

Batteries	Visuospatial Processing
Bexley-Maudsley Automated Psychological Screening	Line Bisection Test
First Mate Perceptual Skill Builder	Search for the Odd Shape
	Searching for Shapes
Memory	Shape Matching
Free Recall	Visual Scanning Test
Memory Span	
Randt Memory Test	*Attention*
Sequence Recall	Digit–Digit II Task
Self-administered Free Recall	Complex Attention Rehabilitation
Word Memory Test	Visual Attention Task
Triplet Recall Task	
	Problem Solving
	Wisconsin Card Sorting Task

Note: From Krug (1988).

used for research and clinical purposes. Krug (1988) describes 445 computer-based products of which 8% are classified as being neuropsychological in their primary application. Most of these are scoring and interpretational programs (see Table 1); examples of programs for computer-administered tests are given in Table 2. Krug (1988) provides an appropriate warning to those using the manual; he writes

> those who are already familiar with computerized assessment know there is considerable variance in the quality of the products currently available. Many are well crafted and designed by knowledgeable professionals. Some are well packaged and marketed aggressively but lack substance and quality. Others are not even well packaged!

Below, consideration is given to some of the potential advantages and problems inherent in computerized testing.

Advantages

Precise Timing

Computerized administration allows for precise time control over both stimulus presentation and response measurement. Timing tests is generally very simple on a computer as most machines have a built-in clock. Control of other dimensions of the stimulus material is possible (e.g., the position, velocity, or acceleration of a point on a visual display).

Experimenter Effects

Experimenter effects are at least partly eliminated. Boredom and fatigue can arise from sitting through a repetitive series of operations, which can increase the risk of administration and scoring errors.

> Nothing is dull, monotonous, boring, routine or too mundane for a computer.... Minute after minute, hour after hour, day after day, week after week, they vigorously pay close attention to detail and adhere to the finest points of standardised testing (Cohen et al. 1988).

Interference from the amount and quality of interaction by the experimenter is prevented. Taylor (1983) argues that, although conventional tests have manuals that specify correct testing procedures, this method of standardization is inadequate in several ways.

> 1. Testers often inadvertently or deliberately depart from the procedures laid down in the manual.

2. The tone of the [tester's] voice can either emphasise or de-emphasise a point.

3. Gestures and idiosyncrasies on the part of the tester can affect the quality of instruction.

4. The tester may rush through the instructional material leaving some of the testees behind or be so meticulous and slow that he bores some of them.

5. Test manuals often omit contingency procedures for certain eventualities. A surprising number of tests do not even have manuals.

6. Tests are sometimes timed with insufficient care.

Computerized testing, Taylor believes, overcomes all of these problems.

Such experimenter effects become of greater concern in longitudinal designs, particularly where repeat assessments take place over several years. Staff turnover may result in follow-up assessments being undertaken by different personnel. Demographic details, such as age and sex of the test administrator, may influence the level of performance of a patient.

Manpower Savings

Computers can save considerable time and release human testers for other duties. This being the case the potential exists for expansion of services and reduction of waiting lists (Beaumont 1981). In their evaluation of computerized assessment, Beaumont and French (1987) also included estimations from clinicians of time saved as a consequence of the automated procedures. Figures given included an average of 10 minutes per test to approximately a 60% reduction in total time.

Improved Scoring

Accuracy and speed of scoring can be improved. Hartman (1986) highlights the potential for the reduction of measurement error from paper-and-pencil measures. Computers also offer a means of systematically gathering and accessing normative databases that transcend the capacities of human test administrators. These factors should enhance test reliability and minimize experimenter bias.

Increased Range of Scores

Computerized testing can produce a range of scores, which is perceived by some as a major advantage. It allows for more data on the subject's performance, which may assist in determining which factors are represented in the final score of the test (Jones & Weinman 1973, Sampson 1983, Taylor 1983).

Sampson suggests that computers can be programmed to identify random response patterns, testee fatigue, and changes in response latency for items that comprise a particular scale or content.

Increased Research Opportunities

Computerized neuropsychological assessment affords considerable opportunities for research. The computer has unique data collection and storage capabilities making research possible that was previously prohibitively difficult or impossible; for instance, the construction of new types of tasks based on models of human information processing (Taylor 1983).

Adaptive Testing Opportunities

Microcomputers make criterion reference testing a feasible alternative to normative based testing. This facility for adaptive testing is emphasized by many (Sampson 1983; Taylor 1983; Weiss 1985). Test taking becomes an interactive process with the directions and items administered varying as a function of the test taker's response. As in traditional testing, the test might begin with some practice items. However, the computer may not permit the test taker to continue on to the test proper until practice items have been responded to in a satisfactory manner or evidence has been acquired that he or she understands the test procedure. If items are ordered according to level of difficulty the program can leap forward to implement most of the testing at the ability level of the individual. The principles of adaptive testing were first applied in the construction of the Binet intelligence test in the early 1900s (Weiss 1985).

Test Administration Without Training

It has been argued that computerized testing is easier to carry out than traditional testing because examiners do not require training in test administration, which is automatically undertaken by computer. For this reason, monitoring computer test administration can be undertaken by technicians, nurses, and other personnel (Denner 1977).

Well Accepted by Users

Investigations into reactions of subjects to computerized testing has generally found very positive responses. Taylor (1983) writes "the evidence indicates that people enjoy being tested on computers and have little difficulty adapting to this type of test." Some report computerized assessment is more acceptable and less threatening than traditional face-to-face experience (Gedye & Miller 1969; Jones & Weinman 1973).

Wide Application

Computer testing can have wide application, with ingenious use of peripherals such as voice recognition, touch panels, or eye-tracking systems (Kennedy et al. 1987), so that sensory and physical limitations may be bypassed. Wilson et al. (1982) developed a dental plate activated by the tongue as the mechanism for test response by test takers who lack the capacity for speech or limb control.

Rehabilitation Potential

Computerized assessment enables the design of intrinsically motivating tests (Kennedy et al. 1987) by making it possible to give subjects feedback on their performance according to preset criteria immediately after each response item. This instant feedback has potential for rehabilitation.

Disadvantages

Cost

Computers are expensive although hardware costs have significantly dropped. Software and maintenance costs must also be considered (Bird 1981). Software can be expensive. The alternative is to self-program. However, this too can be expensive in terms of man hours, particularly if new programming languages need to be acquired. Costs involved may make widespread computer use prohibitive for some institutions.

Loss of Direct Observational Data

Computer test administration deprives the experimenter of the opportunity of direct patient observation (Bird 1981). Unexpected behavioral responses frequently provide the material for later experimental work. One way to get around this is to have closed-circuit television. Loss of direct observation by experienced clinicians may be considered less of a problem where neuropsychological assessment is technician based (Berent 1980).

Inadequate Provision for Human Factors

Sampson (1983) notes that computer test administration often makes inadequate provision for human factors such as response errors and failure to follow or understand the instructions given. Thus depressing the wrong response button can arise through carelessness. This is more of a problem if the individual is required to utilize the traditional keyboard where anyone with poor dexterity is particularly susceptible to making such errors.

Inadequate Reliability Data

Many of the available automated tests have not been well evaluated as regards their psychometric properties. Reliability studies are few and often based on small numbers.

Inadequate Validity Data

Validity is also a concern. Automated tests are often derived from existing ones. However, often there is no test of comparability (Hofer & Green 1985). Not all tests can be be automated so as to be psychometrically parallel to the standard version. The scores may be comparable but equivalence can only be determined on the basis of a formal study expressly designed to examine this. It is conceivable that two computer-based versions of the same test—one where instructions appear on the screen and one via a speech simulator, may not yield equivalent scores. Indeed, such findings were reported by Beaumont and French (1987). Hartman (1986) emphasizes that computerized assessment devices require validation in that format with the generation of new norms.

The issue of validity must also be raised where automated interpretation of the objective test result is provided. Indeed, some programs have report-writing facilities so that a written report is based on a number of computerized measures. Matarazzo (1986) expressed the reservation that untrained purchasers of computerized psychological tests are easily beguiled into believing "she/he now possesses a low cost in-house clinical psychologist who will provide a timely, highly objective valid assessment." There seems to be justifiable concern that the novelty and unquestioned credibility of the computer in some peoples' minds may mask the inadequacies of the interpretations provided. Decision making by an experienced neuropsychologist is complex, and includes consideration of multiple determinants of neuropsychological performance (Adams & Heaton 1985).

Malfunctions Can Occur

Microcomputers are subject to malfunction. Mechanical failure could disrupt an ongoing research program, particularly if parts need replacing or repairing. Beaumont and French (1987) note that the hardware in their study proved to be reliable with only "minor failures causing brief disruption at two sites."

Computerized scoring routines are not infallible. Errors may exist but be difficult to detect. Scoring of programs needs to be regularly updated and modified as relevant information appears in the testing literature.

Inaccessibility of Some Areas of Cognitive Functioning

Some aspects of neuropsychological assessment are less accessible via computer (Adams & Heaton 1985). For example, computers are biased toward the visual modality and vertical presentation. The quality of the image can be limiting, although significant improvements are continually occurring. Expressive language functions and praxis are not readily assessed via computer.

Not Portable

Most microcomputer systems are not easily portable, although over the years there has been a significant reduction in size. Popper et al. (1988) describe a study involving self-administration of cognitive tests via a pocket computer during 30 days of military service.

Biased Toward the Literate

Computerized neuropsychological assessment is biased toward the literate (Taylor 1983). Instructions are often given in written form. Some argue that this problem will be overcome with the development of "speaking" terminals. However, it is difficult to envisage low-cost microcomputers with requisite peripherals coping with a patient asking for repetition or allowing for patients mishearing instructions.

Applications to Epilepsy

Neuropsychological assessment has a long and established role in the evaluation of persons with epilepsy (Trimble & Thompson 1986; Dodrill 1988; Hermann this volume). Thus it seems timely to discern if some consensus can be achieved as to how these techniques can be most profitably employed. Here, I present my personal views regarding the role of computerized testing in epilepsy. Other viewpoints can be found in this volume and elsewhere (Moerland et al. 1986, 1988; Alpherts 1987).

Computerized neuropsychological assessment primarily offers a means of extending the range of neuropsychological assessment techniques rather than replacing traditional methods. Existing evidence considered above indicates that traditional measures when adapted for computer administration are not the same tests, and that in certain areas neuropsychological assessment does not readily lend itself to computerization. Further, the complexities of clinical neuropsychological decision making make me dubious about computerized test interpretations. Computerized assessment measures offer the means of developing novel methods with specific application and as such have enormous research potential. Adaptive testing opportunities afforded by computerized test delivery have possibilities for broadening individual assessments and for developing rehabilitation programs.

One example of the successful use of computerized adaptive testing is in the area of transitory cognitive impairment (TCI) (Binnie 1988; Rugland et al.

1989; also chapters presented in this volume). Understanding of the phenomenon of TCI has greatly increased through the application of microcomputerized assessment. Traditional neuropsychological techniques can only be correlated with the EEG in a very unsatisfactory way. By interfacing the microcomputer with the EEG, signals and responses can be precisely correlated (Moreland et al. 1988). It has to be borne in mind that such computerized systems requiring on-line EEG recording are costly and for this reason are likely to remain the province of specialist centers. Where on-line EEG facilities are not available, it could be argued that traditional test administration by an experienced clinician is more likely to detect subtle seizures by careful observation and that computerized assessment in such a setting may miss or more likely misconstrue such events.

Computerized test administration offers advantages over many existing traditional tests particularly when repeat testing is required and intertest intervals are short. Advantages include the ability to generate parallel versions and the improved standardization in terms of test delivery and scoring. Andrewes and colleagues (1990) described a computerized technique that is being developed for presurgical neuropsychological evaluation. These authors have developed a verbal and visuospatial recognition memory task. The tests were administered to patients via a microcomputer on 8 interictal trials, 2 postictal trials, and again on two occasions one and two weeks following surgery. Computerized delivery enabled standard administration and accurate measurement of responses. Computerized scoring was also able to handle the complex statistical procedures necessary, including the need to equate the verbal and nonverbal versions for difficulty.

Potential for computerized neuropsychological assessment exists in the area of psychopharmacologic investigations. Already such techniques have been employed to assess effects of antidepressants, benzodiazepines and other compounds (review Cull & Trimble 1987). At the National Hospitals in the late 1970s we were involved in designing and conducting cognitive assessments of patients undergoing a variety of medication changes. Before embarking on such studies considerable time was devoted to selecting appropriate neuropsychological measures. Problems were noted with traditional techniques, most notably, no or few parallel versions, lack of precision in test administration, and lack of sensitivity to more subtle cognitive changes, such as mental slowing reported by patients with epilepsy. For this reason, automated test administration was chosen for the studies; these have been described in detail elsewhere (Thompson & Trimble 1982). On completion of a series of studies it seemed that microcomputers offered the next logical step in monitoring effects of antiepileptic drugs. "For increased efficiency and perhaps sensitivity, computerized psychological testing would seem to offer considerable advantages over the equipment employed in these studies" (Thompson 1981). Others have recognized the potential of computerized testing in the monitoring of antiepileptic drugs (Martinius 1980; Tomlinson et al. 1982; Aldenkamp et al. 1987; Alpherts et al. 1987).

Studies at the National Hospitals undertaken in the 1980s did involve computerized neuropsychological test administration. The battery of tests developed included measures of simple reaction time, sustained attention, mental arithmetic, recognition memory for faces and words, and a decision-making task. Using this computerized battery, Cull and Trimble (1989) have reported improvement in test performance following drug reduction and detrimental effects of drug increases in children with epilepsy. Deficits in association with clonazepam and clobazam administration were also reported in a study with healthy volunteers (Cull & Trimble 1985). However, Cull and Trimble (1987) have reported that their battery of computerized tests was subject to practice effects. Whether this was due to the tests themselves or to a change in computer–subject interaction they were unable to say.

Current work being undertaken at the National Hospitals' Assessment Centre for Epilepsy on drug effects includes both traditional paper-and-pencil measures and computerized test administration. By combining both techniques it is hoped to assess the acceptability and usefulness of the two types of measures. The computerized tests have been drawn from the FePsy battery (Moerland et al. 1986, 1988). These computerized tests were preferred to "home grown" measures because they are already being used in a number of European countries and some success in monitoring drug effects has been reported (Aldenkamp et al. 1987; Alpherts et al. 1987). In the future, employment of identical computerized systems will result in less intercenter variability in testing procedures and administration, which will make viable direct comparison of results between centers. In this way rapid accumulation of information of patients having comparable drug changes will be possible.

Controversy reigns concerning the application and interpretation of findings from computerized test administration and particularly regarding the interpretation of reaction time data. One issue is whether changes in processing time in milliseconds reported following drug reductions (e.g., Thompson & Trimble 1982) have any bearing on functioning in everyday life (Dodrill 1988).

> An area of concern is whether a change in psychological test performance has any meaning for cognitive functioning in various daily activities. If following drug changes a patient can recall three more words or make decisions about the color of an object 300 milliseconds faster, does this really have any significant influence on his or her cognitive efficiency? Decision making and memory may well be different when embedded in natural activity than when they are measured in laboratory tasks (Thompson 1981).

However, it is possible that demands on memory, attention, and decision making are greater at work, school, and in social situations than in the very controlled laboratory conditions and that changes in reaction time noted in the laboratory may underestimate changes in everyday life.

We concluded that certain anticonvulsant drugs appeared to induce cognitive slowing (Thompson & Trimble 1982). Alternatively, the observed slowing represents a motor rather than a cognitive phenomenon (Dodrill & Troupin 1991). Computerized testing is well suited to exploring the cognitive slowing hypothesis.

Conclusion

Computerized assessment has a role in the neuropsychological evaluation of persons with epilepsy. Such techniques can be integrated with existing measures and provide a means of extending and refining our assessment measures. Certain areas lend themselves more readily to the computerized approaches, most notably anticonvulsant drug monitoring.

References

Acker WA. Computerized approach to psychological screening—the Bexley-Maudsley automated psychological screening and the Bexley-Maudsley category sorting test. *International Journal of Man-Machine Studies*, 1983, 18:361–369.

Adams KM & Heaton RK. Automated interpretation of neuropsychological test data. *Journal of Consulting and Clinical Psychology*, 1985, 53:790–802.

Aldenkamp AP, Alpherts WCJ, Moerland MC, Ottevanger N & Van Parijs JAP. Controlled release carbamazepine: Cognitive side effects in patients with epilepsy. *Epilepsia*, 1987, 28:507–514.

Alpherts WCJ. (1987). Computers as a technique for neuropsychological assessment in epilepsy. In: AP Aldenkamp, WCJ Alpherts, H Meinardi & G Stores (eds.), *Education and epilepsy* (pp. 101–110). Lisse: Swets and Zeitlinger.

Alpherts WCJ, Aldenkamp AP & Moerland MC. CGP 11.952: An experimental benzodiazepine derivate. Effect on cognitive functioning in patients with epilepsy. *Progress in Neuro-Psychopharmacology and Biological Psychiatry*, 1987, 11:673–678.

Andrewes DG, Puce A & Bladin PF. Post-ictal recognition memory predicts laterality of temporal lobe seizure focus: Comparison with postoperative data. *Neuropsychologia*, 1990, 28:957–967.

Beaumont JG. (1981). Report. Microcomputer aided assessment in psychiatric and neurologic states. Phase 1. London: Department of Health and Social Security.

Beaumont JG & French CC. A clinical field study of eight automated psychometric procedures: The Leicester/DHSS project. *International Journal of Man-Machine Studies*, 1987, 26:661–682.

Berent S. (1980). Psychological assessment in epilepsy: A case illustration. In: B Kulig, H Meinardi & G Stores (eds.), *Epilepsy and behavior '79* (pp. 25–49). Lisse: Swets and Zeitlinger.

Binnie CD. (1988). Seizures, EEG discharges and cognition. In: MR Trimble & EH Reynolds (eds.), *Epilepsy, behavior and cognitive function* (pp. 45-50). Chichester: John Wiley and Sons.

Bird RJ. (1981). *The computer in experimental psychology*. London: Academic Press.

Cohen RJ, Montague P, Nathanson LS, Swerdlik ME & Cohen RJ. (1988). *Psychological testing: An introduction to tests and measurement*. Mountainview, CA: Mayfield Publishing.

Cull CA & Trimble MR. (1985). Anticonvulsant benzodiazepines and performance. In: I Hindmarch, PD Stonier & MR Trimble (eds.), *Clobazam: Human psychopharmacology and clinical applications* (pp. 121-128). Royal Society of Medicine, International Congress and Symposium Series, no. 74. London: Royal Society of Medicine.

Cull CA & Trimble MR. (1987). Automated testing and psychopharmacology. In: I Hindmarch & PD Stonier (eds.), *Human psychopharmacology* (vol. 1) (pp. 113-153). Chichester: John Wiley and Sons.

Cull C & Trimble MR. (1989). Effects of anticonvulsant medications on cognitive functioning in children with epilepsy. In: B Hermann & M Seidenberg (eds.), *Childhood epilepsies: Neuropsychological, psychosocial and intervention aspects* (pp. 83-103). Chichester: John Wiley and Sons.

Denner SA. Automated psychological testing: A review. *British Journal of Social and Clinical Psychology*, 1977, 16:175-179.

Dodrill CB. (1988). Neuropsychology. In: J Laidlaw, A Richens & J Oxley (eds.), *A textbook of epilepsy* (pp. 406-410), 3d ed. Edinburgh: Churchill Livingstone.

Dodrill CB & Troupin AS. Neuropsychological effects of carbamazepine and phenytoin: A reanalysis. *Neurology*, 1991, 41:141-143.

Elithorn A, Lunzer M & Winman J. Cognitive deficits associated with chronic hepatic encephalopathy and their response to levodopa. *Journal of Neurology, Neurosurgery and Psychiatry*, 1975, 38:794-798.

Elithorn A, Mornington S & Stavrou A. Automated psychological testing: Some principles and practice. *International Journal of Man-Machine Studies*, 1982, 17: 247-263.

Elwood DL & Griffin HR. Individual intelligence testing without the examiner: Reliability of an automated method. *Journal of Consulting and Clinical Psychology*, 1972, 38:9-14.

Evans C. (1979). *The mighty micro*. Sevenoaks: Hodder and Stoughton.

Fowler RD. Landmarks in computer-assisted psychological assessment. *Journal of Consulting and Clinical Psychology*, 1985, 53:748-759.

Gedye JL & Miller E. The automation of psychological assessment. *International Journal of Man-Machine Studies*, 1969, 1:237-262.

Gilberstadt H, Lushene R & Buegel B. Automated assessment of intelligence. The TAPAC test battery and computerized report writing. *Perceptual and Motor Skills*, 1976, 43:627-635.

Hartman DE. Artificial intelligence or artificial psychologist? Conceptual issues in clinical microcomputer use. *Professional Psychology: Research and Practice*, 1986, 17:528-534.

Hofer PJ & Green BF. The challenge of competence and creativity in computerized psychological testing. *Journal of Consulting and Clinical Psychology*, 1985, 53:826–838.

Jones D & Weinman J. (1973). Computer based psychological testing. In: A Elithorn & D Jones (eds.), *Artificial and human thinking* (pp. 83–93). Amsterdam: Elsevier Scientific.

Kennedy RS, Wilkes RL, Dunlap WP & Kurtz LP. Development of an automated performance test system for environmental and behavioral toxicology studies. *Perceptual and Motor Skills*, 1987, 65:947–962.

Krug SE (ed.). (1988). *Psychware sourcebook*, 3d ed. Kansas City: Test Corporation of America.

Martinius J. (1980).A programmed system for testing performance in children. In: B Kulig, H Meinardi & G Stores (eds.), *Epilepsy and behavior '79* (pp. 172–176). Lisse: Swets and Zeitlinger.

Matarazzo JD. Computerized clinical psychological test interpretation: Unvalidated plus all mean and no sigma. *American Psychologist*, 1986, 41:14–24.

Moerland MC, Aldenkamp AP & Alpherts WCJ. A neuropsychological test battery for the Apple IIE. *International Journal of Man-Machine Studies*, 1986, 25:453–466.

Moerland MC, Aldenkamp AP & Alpherts WCJ. (1988). Computerized psychological testing in epilepsy. In: FJ Maarse, LJM Mulder, WPB Sjouw & AE Akkerman (eds.), *Computers in psychology: Methods, instrumentation and psychodiagnostics* (pp. 157–164). Lisse: Swets and Zeitlinger.

Popper R, Dragsback H, Siegal SF & Hirsch E. Use of pocket computers for self-administration of cognitive tests in the field. *Behavior Research, Methods, Instruments and Computers*, 1988, 20:481–484.

Rugland AL, Bjornaes H & Henrikesen O. Individual cognitive effects of subclinical EEG discharges in three patients with epilepsy. Paper presented at the 18th International Congress, New Delhi, India, October 1989.

Sampson JP. Computer assisted testing and assessment: Current status and implications for the future. *Measurement and Evaluation in Guidance*, 1983, 15:293–299.

Taylor TR. Computerised testing. *South African Journal of Psychology*, 1983, 13:23–31.

Thompson PJ. The effects of anticonvulsant drugs on healthy volunteers and patients with epilepsy. PhD thesis, University of London, 1981.

Thompson PJ & Trimble MR. Anticonvulsant drugs and cognitive functions. *Epilepsia*, 1982, 23:531–544.

Tomlinson L, Andrewes D, Merrifield E & Reynolds EH. The effects of antiepileptic drugs on cognitive and motor functions. *British Journal of Clinical Practice*, Symposium Supplement, 1982, 18:177–483.

Trimble MR & Thompson PJ (1986). Neuropsychology of epilepsy and its treatment. In: I Grant & KH Adams (eds.), *Neuropsychological assessment of neuropsychiatric disorders* (pp. 321–346). New York: Oxford University Press.

Weiss DJ. Adaptive testing by computer. *Journal of Consulting and Clinical Psychology*, 1985, 53:774–789.

Wilson SL, Thompson JA & Wylie G. Automated psychological testing for the severely physically handicapped. *International Journal of Man-Machine Studies*, 1982, 17:291–296.

4

Validity of Computerized Testing: Patient Dysfunction and Complaints versus Measured Changes

A.P. Aldenkamp, J. Vermeulen, W.C.J. Alpherts,
J. Overweg, J.A.P. Van Parijs
Instituut voor Epilepsiebestrijding 'Meer & Bosch/De Cruquiushoeve'
Heemstede, The Netherlands

N.P.L.G. Verhoeff
Academic Medical Centre, Department of Nuclear Medicine
Amsterdam, The Netherlands

Introduction

In recent years, a substantial amount of research has been carried out on the relationship between cognitive functioning in epilepsy and various epilepsy-related conditions (Kulig et al. 1980; Hermann et al. 1987; Dodrill 1986; Rodin et al. 1986; Trimble & Reynolds 1987; Aldenkamp et al. 1989, 1990a,b). In particular, many studies have established the effects of antiepileptic medication on cognition (Smith et al. 1986; Trimble 1987, 1990). Accordingly, the emphasis in research on antiepileptic drugs has shifted from seizure control to a more comprehensive approach in which the prevention of cognitive side effects is given due attention (Trimble & Reynolds 1987; Aldenkamp & Dodson 1990; Gram 1990).

In clinical practice, however, the opportunities for the assessment of the cognitive functions that are thought to be particularly vulnerable in epilepsy, such as memory and attention, are usually very limited. Therefore, patient complaints suggestive of problems in such areas of functioning often represent the only available evidence of possible cognitive dysfunction. Patient complaints should be taken seriously, of course, if only because they may reflect organic factors such as inadequate serum levels of antiepileptic drugs that may interfere with cognitive functioning and need correction. However, it would be unwise to take all patient complaints that suggest cognitive dysfunction at face value. While some patients may have a clear insight into their own capabilities and failures, others may have a poor understanding of their performance or they may forget past failures. In its most impressive form this phenomenon occurs in certain aphasics or in densely amnestic patients, who have little or no insight into a disorder that is readily apparent to others and that has a dramatic effect in daily life (McGlynn & Schacter 1989). At the other end of the spectrum we may find patients whose cognitive complaints reflect personality factors, perhaps augmented by the stress induced by a chronic condition such as epilepsy.

Thus discrepancies between patient complaints and the outcome of psychological testing of cognitive functions may arise, a situation that, in our experience, occurs fairly regularly in clinical practice. Patients may be "doing better but feeling worse" (cf. *The Lancet*), and vice versa. Of course a divergence between dysfunction as perceived by the patient and as revealed by psychological tests may also be due to inadequacies in the current assessment methods. For example, traditional psychological tests may fail to capture certain types of cognitive dysfunction specific to epilepsy, such as transient cognitive impairment associated with subclinical absences (Thompson & Huppert 1980; Ossetin 1987; Loiseau et al. 1987).

This chapter reviews some of the relevant studies on the relationship between patient complaints and cognitive dysfunction in epilepsy, elaborating some of the points raised in the foregoing.

Prevalence of Cognitive Complaints

Several authors report that persons with epilepsy frequently complain about cognitive deficits. Memory complaints are especially mentioned as a dominant factor in clinical practice (Stores 1981; Loiseau et al. 1982, 1987; Thompson 1989). Nevertheless, exact frequencies of such complaints cannot be found in literature. At best, general indications are provided "people with epilepsy frequently complain of memory disturbance..." (Thompson 1989). Some findings from our own research may give us an indication. During a 3-months' follow-up in an outpatient unit, we included each patient with spontaneous memory complaints in a study in cooperation with the department of nuclear medicine, Amsterdam (Overweg et al. 1990; Verhoeff et al. in press). Of the 153 patients who were seen by the neurologist, 31 (20.2%) had spontaneous memory complaints. All patients in this study had a therapy resistant partial epilepsy.

TABLE 1

Percentage of Patient Complaints in the
"Holmfrid" Multicenter Withdrawal Study[a]

Samples[b]	Epilepsy	Controls
Type of Complaint		
Alertness	13.0[c]	6.0
Concentration	10.7	12.1
Drowsiness	14.5	10.8
Tiredness	*22.8*	9.6
Depression	8.0	2.4
Irritation	18.0	12.1
Aggressiveness	18.0	10.8
Overactive	19.3	19.3
Memory	*22.8*	9.6

Notes: [a] Preliminary results of the multicenter "Holmfrid" withdrawal study (Blennow et al. 1990) after assessment of 83 children. Final results are to be described separately. Values before withdrawal of antiepileptic drug treatment are listed.

[b] The average age of these children was 12.6 at the start of the study (for both groups), the average duration of the epilepsy was 4.7 years (range 2–12 years) and the children were seizure free for an average period of 3 years (range 1–8 years). All children were of normal intelligence.

[c] Values indicate the percentage of patients with complaints, values above 20% are in italics.

As to the type of their complaints, most patients (57%) have subjective retention complaints (problems with long-term recall) or acquisition complaints (difficulties in learning new information). Retrieval complaints (such as the tip of the tongue phenomenon) are only reported in a minority of the patients (7%). This is not in line with other studies on memory loss in elderly patients where retrieval complaints are most often found (Neisser & Herrmann 1978). Moreover, in a study on 80 outpatients with epilepsy, Thompson (1989) found that retrieval problems were predominant.

In a multicenter study, conducted with 10 pediatric centers in Sweden (Blenow et al. 1990), 83 children who were seizure free for at least 1 year and who were on antiepileptic monotherapy, were matched to normal controls and assessed both before and after withdrawal of their drugs.[1] As part of the assessment procedures the subjective memory complaints were evaluated.

---

[1] Preliminary data of the multicenter "Holmfrid" withdrawal study (Blennow et al. 1990) after assessment of 83 children. Final results are to be described separately.

During treatment, 22.8% of the patients had memory complaints. This is significantly more than is found in matched controls where 9.6% of the children have memory complaints. The same difference is found when the self-reports are supplemented with reports of the parents about their children. Table 1 illustrates that beside memory complaints, patients frequently complain about tiredness (italicized values). In other areas less than 20% of the patients complain. An average of 16.5% of the patients have cognitive complaints versus 10.3% of normal controls. Thus cognitive complaints are more frequent in patients with epilepsy than in non-neurological populations. Spontaneous cognitive complaints may be encountered in up to 20% of the patients with epilepsy. Memory complaints are among the most common cognitive complaints, regardless of subgroup.

Patient Complaints and Measured Cognitive Function

Several studies mention discrepancies between patient complaints and the results of cognitive testing (Deyo 1984). This has been discussed since James raised this issue in 1890 and Freud in 1914 (see Herrmann 1982). In epilepsy this dispute has centered around the existence of memory loss in patients with epilepsy (Scott et al. 1967). Thompson (1989) concludes that many patients who complain often perform within normal limits on standardized memory tests. Our own research shows this same tendency and illustrates that the relationships between patient complaints and results of cognitive testing are complex.

In a controlled parallel group study, patient complaints, results of cognitive tests, and a mood rating scale were assessed in matched pairs of patients on carbamazepine (CBZ) and phenytoin (PHT) (Hiltbrunner et al. 1991, in prep.). In each group 9 patients were included. To avoid bias due to treatment allocation, treatment with carbamazepine did not precede treatment with phenytoin and vice versa. Spontaneous patient complaints are observed in 7 of 9 cases in the CBZ group and in 3 of 9 cases in the PHT group.

Results of an administered computerized test battery are listed in Table 2. Only tasks with a speed factor have been included here because most differences between the two drugs have been reported to be related to speed characteristics (Smith et al. 1986; Ossetin 1987; Trimble 1990). The differences between CBZ and PHT are consistent and demonstrate slower reaction times in all tasks for PHT. The obtained slowing in the Complex Visual Searching Task (CVST) illustrates that this is not exclusively caused by motor slowing, as suggested in some recent studies (Dodrill & Temkin 1989; Dodrill & Troupin 1991). An exception is the reaction time for the Binary Choice Task, which is faster in PHT, albeit at the cost of more errors. For motor speed, as measured with the Finger Tapping Task, a reverse relationship has been found (CBZ slower), in line with earlier studies (Trimble & Thompson 1983).

TABLE 2

Patient Complaints versus Measured Cognitive Changes
in Patients on Carbamazepine and Phenytoin:
Results of the Computerized Reaction Time Tests

	CBZ^a	PHT	CBZ^B	PHT^C
Simple Motor Reaction Time				
Auditory stimulus, right hand	228.7 (38.4)	255.1 (90.4)	+	
Auditory stimulus, left hand	218.4 (27.5)	233.4 (58.1)	+	
Visual stimulus, right hand	260.2 (26.2)	283.2 (71.1)	+	
Visual stimulus, left hand	265.5 (27.2)	289.8 (99.3)	+	
Complex Reaction Time				
Binary Choice Reaction Task				
Correct responses	56.6 (2.7)	55.2 (8.6)	+	
Reaction time	441.7 (102.3)	374.2 (130.7)		+
Visual Searching Task				
Reaction time	10.11 (3.0)	12.7 (10.2)	+	
Motor Fluency				
Finger tapping, right hand	56.5 (5.4)	61.8 (7.9)		+
Finger tapping, left hand	50.3 (4.0)	54.3 (8.6)		+

Notes: [a] All patients in the CBZ group were on treatment with a controlled-release preparation (Tegretol-CR). All patients have low serum levels except for 2 patients in the CBZ group with serum levels slightly above 3U μmoL/mL. The groups are matched for education level, seizure type, and epilepsy diagnosis.
[b] CBZ+ = Performance CBZ higher than PHT.
[c] PHT+ = Performance PHT higher than CBZ.

The results of the Profiled Mood States (POMS) mood rating scale (McNair et al. 1971) show a total mood disturbance score (TMD) of 48.0 (SD 10.2) for CBZ (derived from 65 items on a 5-point scale) and 61.0 for PHT (SD 23.2), demonstrating more mood disturbance in the patients on PHT.

The results discussed above are summarized in Table 3 and illustrate that patients on phenytoin complained less about cognitive side effects of their treatment, but actually showed more impairment on cognitive tests and on a mood-rating scale than patients on carbamazepine.

TABLE 3

Patient Complaints versus Results of Cognitive Tests and a
Mood Rating Scale in Patients on Carbamazepine and Phenytoin

	Carbamazepine	*Phenytoin*
Subjective (spontaneous) complaints	severe disturbance	mild disturbance
Results cognitive (reaction time) tests	mild disturbance	severe disturbance
Results POMS mood rating scale	mild disturbance	severe disturbance

For a partial explanation of these discrepancies we may use the concept of "unawareness of cognitive impairment." "Unawareness" is also found in, for example, amnestic or aphasic patients who have little insight into their own disability (McGlynn & Schacter 1989). As a consequence, these patients may overestimate their capacities to remember information or to process language adequately (Shimamura & Squire 1986). Unawareness for motor and mental slowing may explain the results for the PHT group in our study. Consequently, we may underestimate the seriousness and even the very existence of cognitive handicaps in some patients with epilepsy.

On the other hand, complaints may lead to overestimation of dysfunction, because—in patients with epilepsy—complaints may be erroneously interpreted as manifestations of neurological impairment. Thompson (1989) reports over-estimation of the significance of complaints in patients with epilepsy as a consequence of negative self-evaluation.

Although 22.8% of the patients with epilepsy included in the aforementioned multicenter withdrawal trial (Blennow et al. 1990) had subjective memory complaints, the average scores on the memory tests did not diverge significantly from the scores obtained in the normal controls. Only a minority of the patients may be considered as scoring below average. This implies that, in this group, complaints can be confirmed in only a limited number of patients. It should be noted that all patients in this group were seizure free for at least 1 year. Therefore these results may not be valid for other subgroups of patients with epilepsy.

In another study, patients were referred to us for memory assessment as part of the screening for a trial with an experimental psychotropic drug (oxiracetam: 4-hydroxy-2-oxo-pyrrolidine-acetamide, a pyrrolidinone derivative structurally related to a cyclic form of gamma-amino-beta-hydroxybutyric acid) with potential positive effects on memory function (Aldenkamp et al. 1991). All patients had an active form of partial epilepsy and most were on polytherapy. Among the 75 patients with chronic memory complaints who were included in the pretrial screening, 20 (26.7%) were without psychometrically confirmed memory impairment. In this particular group, patients tended to score high on depression and anxiety scales and to express somatic complaints.

In the collaborative study with the department of nuclear medicine, Amster-dam (Overweg et al. 1990; Verhoeff et al. in press) patients were selected who had chronic spontaneous memory complaints. Memory impairment, as estab-lished with cognitive testing was found in 82.1% of the patients, revealing a discrepancy of approximately 20% between patient complaints and measured cognitive impairment.

These findings illustrate that self-reports of patients with epilepsy may have limited reliability and that the use of cognitive complaints in clinical practice perpetuates the risk of using inaccurate estimates of cognitive disability. Some patients may be satisfied with their treatment, despite demonstrable side effects, while others may have serious complaints despite normal scores on cognitive tests. To summarize our own findings with respect to this latter factor: despite chronic memory complaints, we found no indication of memory impairment in about 20% of the patients with active epilepsies. This discrepancy may be greater in patients with seizure remission.

Methods for Self-Assessment:
Spontaneous Complaints versus Standardized Inventories

A common approach to the problem of discrepancies between patient complaints and results of cognitive tests is to employ questionnaires or inventories (Sarason et al. 1978). The rationale behind this approach is that spontaneous complaints may not be consistent and lack structure. Questionnaires aim at systematic evaluations of individuals' beliefs about their performance (Herrmann 1982), that may reflect cognitive performance. Questionnaires have the additional advantage of being a simple method to survey a large number of cognitive phenomena, some of which might otherwise go undetected (Neisser & Herrmann 1978). If evidence could be found for these assumptions, then the ideal of assessing cognitive performance in natural circumstances would be attained. However, several studies have failed to find correlations between questionnaires and cognitive tests (Broadbent et al. 1982). This may have been caused by the fact that unawareness of cognitive failure may also affect self-rating in questionnaires. Responding to a questionnaire is in itself a memory task (Sunderland et al. 1983). Bennet-Levy et al. (1980) studied 58 temporal lobectomy patients; no correlations were found between self-ratings and memory tests. An extensive review by Herrmann (1982) illustrates that memory beliefs, as measured by questionnaires, are generally not correlated with scores on cognitive tests.

To date this issue has been addressed as it relates to epilepsy in only a limited number of studies. Thompson (1989) did not obtain a relationship between a standard interview and a series of memory tests, with the exception of a story recall test. Our own data from the collaborative study with the department of nuclear medicine, Amsterdam, point in the same direction (Overweg et al. 1990; Verhoeff et al. in press). Using a standardized memory questionnaire, combined with visual analog scaling and a checklist technique, a large discrepancy was found between the results of this questionnaire and spontaneous memory complaints. Whereas all patients have spontaneous memory complaints (as a consequence of the inclusion criteria), only 67.9% report memory complaints on the questionnaire. Because 82.1% of the patients score below average on cognitive tests, this suggests that spontaneous complaints may overestimate the incidence of actual impairment; a standardized questionnaire may underestimate the incidence. Although no significant correlations were found between type of spontaneous complaints and type of memory disorder, a significant correlation was obtained between type of memory impairment and questionnaire-based complaints: patients with global memory impairment have more complaints. Moreover, these patients report forgetting names as their main problem.

Generally speaking, when cognitive tasks are used that closely mimic real-life skills, the relationship between self-ratings on questionnaires and on cognitive tests are stronger (Bennet-Levy et al. 1980). The relationship that is found between memory complaints and a test for story recall is an example of this (Thompson 1989). Some approaches try to upgrade the reliability of questionnaires by the use of diaries, or by comparing the results with spouse ratings. Indeed, Sunderland and coworkers (1983), studying head-injured patients, reported significant correlations between some of their memory tests and spouse ratings.

Relationship Between Scores on Cognitive Tests and Epileptic Conditions

Patients with epilepsy often believe that their cognitive problems are caused mainly by the drugs they take and not by other factors, such as the seizures. For example, in the aforementioned multicenter withdrawal study (Blennow et al. 1990) the majority of patients with subjective complaints consider these to be drug effects.

Although the central side effects of antiepileptic drugs (AED) are well documented (Trimble 1987, 1990), the issue of the relative contribution of AED therapy compared to other epilepsy-related conditions is still open. Seizure type and frequency are probably important factors (Dodrill 1986) and are complicated by other factors, such as seizure duration (Rodin et al. 1986), and etiology (Dam 1990). There is evidence that the site of the epileptogenic focus may be a crucial factor, especially in explaining type and severity of observed memory disorders. Memory disorders are often found in temporal lobe epilepsy (Hermann et al. 1987). Verbal and visuospatial memory loss are more often associated with an epileptogenic focus in the left and right hemisphere respectively (Ladavas & Umilta 1979; Binnie et al. 1987; Loiseau et al. 1987). The evidence for lateralization of dysfunction has been confirmed to some extent in the course of preoperative WADA testing (Sylfvenius et al. 1984) and in postoperative follow-up studies (Ojemann & Dodrill 1985).

In the collaborative study with the department of nuclear medicine, Amsterdam (Overweg et al. 1990; Verhoeff et al. in press), we studied the relationship between type of memory impairment and neurofunctional factors. A 21-channel EEG was recorded both during cognitive testing and during a Tc-99M-HMPAO Single Photon Emission Computerized Tomography (SPECT). On the same day a CT scan was performed. None of the epilepsy-related factors (seizure type, seizure frequency, type of epilepsy, age at onset of the seizures, type of antiepileptic treatment) could be related directly to severity or type of memory impairment (classified into the categories "global," "verbal," and "nonverbal"). Although, for the type of antiepileptic treatment this may have been caused by the overrepresentation of CBZ in our sample, our findings are in line with the study by Loiseau and coworkers (1982) who found that neither type of epilepsy, frequency of the seizures, duration of the illness, nor medication could account for memory impairment in 200 adults with epilepsy. Remarkably, no significant relationship was found in this study between EEG focus localization and severity of measured memory impairment. This also holds for the subgroup of patients with bilateral foci who showed the same scores as patients with a unilateral (left- or right-sided) foci. This is in accord with other studies that reported no consistent relationship between memory impairment and lateralization of EEG focus (Hermann et al. 1987). Most areas with hypoperfusion on the SPECT were found in the group with global (severe) amnesia, typically with a right frontal localization. CT scan abnormalities were predominantly found in the same group, however, with a right-sided parietal localization. An unanticipated finding was that the majority of temporal CT and SPECT lesions were found in the group with relatively better memory performance. The findings in this study are in contrast to a Xe-133 SPECT study of 50 patients with partial epilepsy, that yielded a significant correlation between lateralization of areas with hypoperfusion and verbal versus figural memory impairment. This relationship was weaker for the frontal lesions than for temporal lesions (Homan et al. 1989). The differences between the studies may be due to the use of different neuropsychological testing methods and to the differences in SPECT technique.

The relationship between hypoperfusion in the frontal lobe and memory impairment may well be one of the reasons for our failure to obtain significant correlations between type and severity of patient complaints and the results of cognitive tests. Unawareness has been reported, especially as it relates to frontal-lobe pathology, in several cognitive syndromes (Jarho 1973; Shimamura & Squire 1986). By contrast, patients with temporal lesions reportedly have more insight into their dysfunction (Bennet-Levy et al. 1980).

Cognitive Assessment Procedures: Measured Cognitive Changes

Obviously, any failure to find a correlation between the cognitive complaints and performance on cognitive tests may simply reflect inadequacies of the tests. The demands placed on memory in everyday life, for example, may or may not be adequately covered by the tasks commonly employed in a psychological laboratory. After all, the neuropsychological tests typically used in epilepsy research tend to be selected on the basis of their ability to detect brain damage or to provide information regarding localization and lateralization of lesions (Ossetin 1987). The ecological validity, that is, the validity in real-life situations, of such tests is open to question (Thompson 1989). Thus, a patient may rightly complain "having trouble remembering things," but his or her problem eludes detection with psychologists' standard repertory of tests if these do not tap the specific aspect of memory the patient is complaining about (Herrmann 1982). An example would be that most standard clinical memory testing involves fairly short retention intervals (i.e., minutes to hours) (Guilford 1971). Retention and forgetting over the long term, as in a person's own memory for long-past events, is obviously much more difficult to test even though a technique involving memory of public events has been devised (Squire et al. 1975).

In addition to such general problems regarding the ecological validity of traditional cognitive tests, the assessment of cognitive functioning in epilepsy poses specific problems. Timing factors appear to be important for explaining cognitive dysfunction in epilepsy (Schwab 1939; Gaillard 1980; Ossetin 1987), sometimes requiring a measurement precision in milliseconds (Alpherts 1987). Side effects of antiepileptic drugs need to be measured with sufficient accuracy to detect the effects of rapid fluctuations in serum levels on cognitive function (Aldenkamp et al. 1987). Correlating EEG parameters with psychological performance requires precise timing of stimulus and response (e.g., in detecting transient cognitive impairment) (Binnie et al. 1987). Traditional psychological

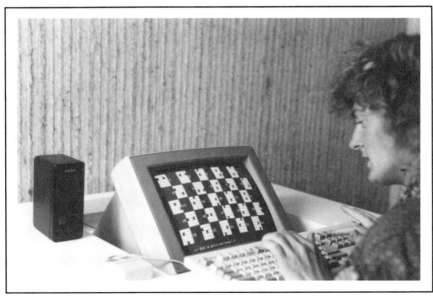

FIGURE 1
Standardized setting for computerized assessment.

instruments may not be entirely adequate for such purposes (for example, see the discussions in Dodrill 1978; Loiseau et al. 1987; Alpherts 1987; Dodrill & Temkin 1989; Dodrill & Troupin 1991) and may thus fail to detect genuine dysfunction underlying a patient's complaint.

Such considerations prompted us to develop a system of automated psychological testing—FePsy (Moeland et al. 1986, 1988; Alpherts 1987; Alpherts & Aldenkamp 1990; Aldenkamp et al. 1990b). The tests can be run on any MSDOS computer and cover such cognitive domains as information processing, memory, vigilance, attention and planning functions. The standardized assessment setting is illustrated in Figure 1. Some examples of results obtained with this system follow.

The Importance of Speed Factors in Epilepsy

Most studies report reaction time in simple motor tasks, but definite slowing in complex reaction tasks (Aldenkamp et al. 1990b). Recently this has come back into debate in research on side effects of AEDs, with a special emphasis on the role of motor speed (Dodrill & Temkin 1989; Meador et al. 1990; Dodrill & Troupin 1991).

Table 4 illustrates that substantial differences between patients with epilepsy and normal controls have been found in complex reaction time tasks, whereas the differences in simple motor reaction time tasks are, in general, moderate.

TABLE 4

Results of Different Reaction Time Tests in Patients with Epilepsy versus Normal Controls

	Adult Subjects[a] Diff. Epilepsy Control[c] (Approximations)	Children[b] Diff. Epilepsy Control (Approximations)
Simple Motor Reaction Time Tests		
Auditory stimului	28.0 msec	2–14 msec[d]
Visual stimuli	25.0 msec	5 msec
Complex Reaction Time Tests		
Binary choice reaction time	95.0 msec	42 msec
Visual searching reaction time	8.4 seconds	2–7 seconds[e]

Notes: [a] Results from a heterogeneous epilepsy sample, referred for clinical assessment. Epilepsy N = 106 (CVST); N = 67 (Tapping Test and Binary Choice Reaction Time Test); N = 609 (Simple Motor Reaction Time Tests) (Alpherts et al. 1985); Controls (normal volunteers) N = 17–103. Norms for simple motor reaction time from Lezak (1976).
[b] Sample: epilepsy N = 94–177 (dependent on tasks); controls N = 68–161; mean reaction time in milliseconds, for the CVST in seconds. Sample description: Alpherts and Aldenkamp (1990).
[c] All results show longer reaction times for patients with epilepsy.
[d] For nondominant and dominant hand respectively.
[e] Mean reaction time for age cohorts 13–18 years.

Other examples suggestive of such general slowing of information processing (mental slowing) have been described elsewhere (Aldenkamp et al. 1990b; Alpherts & Aldenkamp 1990); however, these results have been obtained in patients with epilepsy. Therefore, the differences may be caused by many factors, such as type of AED, type of epilepsy, and etiological factors. Using a large database obtained with this type of assessment, we are currently attempting to isolate some of these factors by analyzing the results for several subgroups.

Detection of Central Side Effects of Antiepileptic Drug Treatment

The detection of central side effects of antiepileptic drugs usually requires repeated measurement and thus offers a particular challenge to our methods of assessment. A patient is tested before and after drug withdrawal, or several times during a day to correlate complaints with the pharmacokinetic properties of a drug (Aldenkamp et al. 1987). This requires efforts to minimize practice effects due to retesting and increase standardization. Computer assessment increases standardization by reducing measurement error variations. Moreover, a computer can easily generate parallel test versions or present items randomly, thus minimizing practice effects. In some of our tests this is achieved by presenting items randomly from a large datapool. The validity of our tasks is currently under investigation. One example will be given as an illustration. One of the objectives of the previously mentioned multicenter withdrawal study (Blennow et al. 1990) was to analyze cognitive side effects of antiepileptic drug treatment.

TABLE 5

Results of Two Complex Reaction Time Tests for Different Drug Groups
in 83 Children with Epilepsy and Matched Controls[a]

Test Assessment	CBZ^b		VPA^c		PHT^d		$Controls^e$	
	1st	*2nd*	*1st*	*2nd*	*1st*	*2nd*	*1st*[f]	*2nd*
Binary Choice Reaction								
Average reaction time	397	371	413	386	465	438	413	368
SD	142	127	155	148	166	108	154	119
Computerized Visual Searching Task								
Average reaction time	15.2	12.9	17.1	14.0	18.9	15.4	15.2	12.2
SD	2.1	1.8	2.8	2.3	3.3	2.2	2.2	1.7

Notes: [a] Preliminary data of the multicenter "Holmfrid" withdrawal study (Blennow et al. 1990) after the assessment of 83 children. Final results are to be described separately.
[b] Carbamazepine, N = 55.
[c] Valproic acid, N = 18.
[d] Phenytoin, N = 8.
[e] Controls, N = 83.
[f] 1st = first assessment, during treatment; 2nd = second assessment after withdrawal of antiepileptic treatment.

Table 5 gives preliminary results of two complex reaction time tests: the Binary Choice Reaction Test and the Computerized Visual Searching Test. These data show that the well-documented effects of phenytoin on mental speed are clearly detected by our instruments. Surprisingly, the observed impairment for PHT persist after drug withdrawal. We are currently analyzing whether this represents a long-term effect of the drug (which would be in line with the data by Gallassi et al. 1988), still measurable after a period of 6 months, or an effect of the underlying epileptic condition.

Electrophysiological Correlates of Fluctuations in Cognitive Performance

The detection of cognitive effects of subclinical absences (Binnie et al. 1987; Kasteleyn-Nolst et al. 1990) obviously requires cognitive assessment procedures with precise response registration that are impossible to achieve without computerized tests. We are currently experimenting with a standard set of tests, assessing different levels of cognitive function, using vigilance tests, memory (recognition) tasks with verbal and nonverbal stimuli, and an information processing task. During this type of simultaneous EEG registration and cognitive testing, the computer continuously provides the EEG with feedback by means

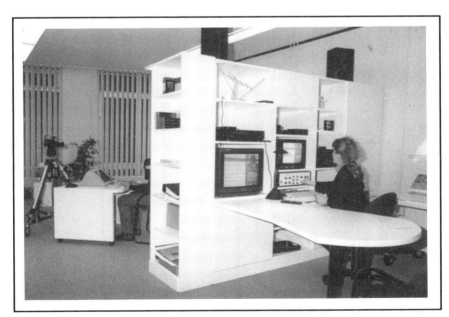

FIGURE 2

Assessment setting for simultaneous EEG recording, videomonitoring, and cognitive testing.

TABLE 6

Results of Cognitive Tests and EEG recordings for 83 Children with Epilepsy[a]

Seizure Type[b]	CVST Number of Errors		Type of AED			EEG Evaluation Bilateral Spike slow wave activity in %	
	1st	2nd		1st	2nd	1st	2nd
Absence	4.3	3.4	CBZ	2.3	1.6	5	9
Tonic-clonic	3.0	2.4	VPA	3.6	3.3	0	39
Complex-partial	2.9	1.9	PHT	1.6	1.2	0	0
Rolandic	1.4	1.2	Controls	2.4	1.6	—	—
Controls	2.4	1.6					

Notes: [a] Preliminary data of the multicenter "Holmfrid" withdrawal study (Blennow et al. 1990) after the assessment of 83 children. Final results are to be described separately.
[b] Four seizure types have been included in this analysis: absence seizures: N = 8, generalized tonic-clonic seizures: N = 15, complex-partial seizures: N = 23, benign form of childhood epilepsy with centro-temporal spikes: N = 26, remaining forms (not included in the table): N = 11.

of an interface device, which gives an output, in real time, of all kinds of parameters, such as response latencies and level of accuracy. Output can be sent to the marker channel, to any other channel, or to an EEG-videoprocessor. Figure 2 illustrates the assessment setting with continuous video monitoring. The value of this assessment for detecting the effects of paroxysmal epileptiform activity in the EEG is illustrated by some preliminary data from the aforementioned multicenter withdrawal study (Blennow et al. 1990).

Table 6 shows the error rate for the Computerized Visual Searching Task (CVST) per seizure type. There is a large difference between the groups, caused by the poorer performance of the group with absence seizures. Closer inquiry revealed that this is caused by the subgroup of patients that used valproic acid at the start of the study. In none of these patients was seizure recurrence observed after withdrawal of the drug. The number of errors on the CVST is also listed by drug group in this table, confirming the higher error rate in the VPA group, both during treatment and after withdrawal of the drug. Independently, the EEGs were analyzed by Dan Elmqvist and his coworkers from the neurophysiological department of Lund University. Table 6 demonstrates that children on valproic acid had an increase of bilateral spike slow-wave activity in the EEG after the drug was withdrawn. This was not accompanied by clinical symptomatology. The lower performance on several of the cognitive tasks for this subgroup may therefore reflect subclinical epileptiform activity. These results do not validate our computerized assessment procedures, but merely illustrate our attempts to increase the potential of our instruments to investigate important clinical issues in epilepsy.

Closing Comments

In contrast to the assessment of physical effects of the epilepsy and of most side effects of antiepileptic treatment, higher-order cognitive functions cannot be adequately assessed by using subjective patient reports or by relying on a clinical impression. Attempts to upgrade the usefulness of patient complaints with questionnaires failed to find significant correlations with patient dysfunction, as indicated by cognitive performance.

An important prerequisite for using patient complaints in clinical practice is to find differential characteristics of patient complaints that are associated with patient dysfunction in epilepsy. Unfortunately, only limited data are available currently. Some studies mention characteristics related to retrieval (tip-of-the-tongue phenomena), whereas our research points to learning or acquisition and to retention complaints. Therefore, only extensive neuropsychological assessment may reveal cognitive impairment, although the ecological validity of these tests is in question.

Considerable effort will be needed to match our assessment procedures to the demands posed by clinical and electrophysiological aspects of epilepsy, which are often subtle or transient but, nevertheless, may have major consequences for daily life functioning.

References

Aldenkamp AP, Alpherts WCJ, Dekker MCA & Overweg J. Neuropsychological aspects in learning disabilities in epilepsy. In: AP Aldenkamp & WE Dodson (eds.), Epilepsy and education; cognitive factors in learning behavior. *Epilepsia*, 1990b (suppl. 4), pp. S9–S20. New York: Raven Press.

Aldenkamp AP, Alpherts WCJ, De Bruïne D & Dekker MJA. Test-retest variability in children with epilepsy—a comparison of WISC-R subtest profiles. *Epilepsy Research*, 1990a, 7:165–172.

Aldenkamp AP, Alpherts WCJ, Meinardi H & Stores G. (1989). *Education and epilepsy*. Swets & Zeitlinger, Lisse/Berwyn (USA).

Aldenkamp AP, Alpherts WCJ, Moerland MC, Ottevanger N & van Parijs JAP. Controlled release carbamazepine: Cognitive side effects in patients with epilepsy. *Epilepsia*, 1987, 28(5):507–514.

Aldenkamp AP & Dodson WE. Epilepsy and education; cognitive factors in learning behavior. *Epilepsia* 31(suppl. 4), 1990. New York: Raven Press.

Aldenkamp AP, Van Wieringen A, Alpherts WCJ, Van Emde Boas W, Haverkort E, De Vries J & Meinardi H. Double-blind placebo-controlled, neuropsychological and neurophysiological investigations with oxiracetam (CGP 21690E) in memory-impaired patients with epilepsy. *Neuropsychobiology*, 1991, 24(2):113–127.

Alpherts WCJ. (1987). Computers as a technique for neuropsychological assessment in epilepsy. In: AP Aldenkamp, WCJ Alpherts, H Meinardi & G Stores (eds.), *Education and epilepsy* (pp. 21–38). Swets & Zeitlinger, Lisse/Berwyn (USA).

Alpherts WCJ & Aldenkamp AP. Computerized neuropsychological assessment in children with epilepsy. In: AP Aldenkamp & WE Dodson (eds.), Epilepsy and education; cognitive factors in learning behavior. *Epilepsia*, 1990 (suppl. 4), pp. S35–S40. New York: Raven Press.

Alpherts WCJ, Aldenkamp AP & Moerland MC. Neuropsychological assessment of cognitive functions in epilepsy. Epilepsy International Congress. Hamburg, 8 September 1985.

Bennet-Levy J, Polkey CE & Powell GE. Self-report of memory skills after temporal lobectomy: The effect of clinical variables. *Cortex*, 1980, 16:543–557.

Binnie CD, Kasteleijn-Nolst Trénité DGA, Smit AM & Wilkins AJ. Interactions of epileptiform EEG discharges and cognition. *Epilepsy Research*, 1987, 1:239–245.

Blennow G, Heijbel J, Sandstedt P & Tonnby B. Discontinuation of antiepileptic drugs in children who have outgrown epilepsy: Effects on cognitive function. In: AP Aldenkamp & WE Dodson (eds.), Epilepsy and education; cognitive factors in learning behavior. *Epilepsia* 31(suppl. 4), 1990, pp. S50–S53. New York: Raven Press.

Broadbent AJ, Coepel JF, Fitzgerald P & Parkes KP. The cognitive failures questionnaire and its correlates. *British Journal of Clinical Psychology*, 1982, 21:1–16.

Dam M. Children with epilepsy: The effect of seizures, syndromes, and etiological factors on cognitive function. In: AP Aldenkamp & WE Dodson (eds.), Epilepsy and education; cognitive factors in learning behavior. *Epilepsia* 31(suppl. 4), 1990, pp S26–S30. New York: Raven Press.

Deyo RA. Measuring functional outcomes in therapeutic trials for chronic disease. *Controlled Clinical Trials*, 1984, 223–240.

Dodrill CB. A neuropsychological battery for epilepsy. *Epilepsia*, 1978, 19:611–623.

Dodrill CB. Correlates of generalized tonic-clonic seizures with intellectual, neuropsychological, emotional and social function in patients with epilepsy. *Epilepsia*, 1986, 27:399–411.

Dodrill CB & Temkin NR. Motor speed is a contaminating factor in evaluating the "cognitive" effects of phenytoin. *Epilepsia*, 1989, 30:453–457.

Dodrill CB & Troupin AS. Neuropsychological effects of carbamazepine and phenytoin: A reanalysis. *Neurology*, 1991, 41:141–143.

Gaillard AWK. (1980). The use of task variables and brain potentials in the assessment of cognitive impairment. In: BM Kulig, H Heinardi & G Stores (eds.), *Epilepsy and behaviour* (pp. 104–111). Amsterdam: Swets & Zeitlinger.

Gallassi, R, Morreale A, Lorusso S, Procaccianti G, Lugaresi E. & Baruzzi A. Comparison of cognitive effects in epileptic patients during monotherapy and withdrawal. *Arch. Neurol.*, 1988, 45:892–894.

Gram, L. (1990). Monitoring drug therapy and side effects. In: M Sillanpaa, SI Johannessen, G Blennow & M Dam (eds.), *Paediatric epilepsy* (pp.53–62). Petersfield: Wrightson Biomedical Publishing Ltd.

Guilford JP. (1971). *The nature of human intelligence*. London: McGraw-Hill.

Hermann BP, Wyler AR, Richey, ET & Rea JM. Memory function and learning ability in patients with complex partial seizures of temporal lobe origin. *Epilepsia*, 1987, 28:547–554.

Herrmann DJ. Know thy memory: The use of questionnaires to assess and study memory. *Psychological Bulletin*, 1982, 92(2):434–452.

Hiltbrunner B, Joyce CRB & Aldenkamp AP. A pilot study to investigate methods of quality of life assessment in epilepsy. Trial Plan TE/QLI. Ciba Geigy, Medical Department, Basel, Switzerland.

Homan RW, Paulman RG, Devous MD, Walker P, Jennings LW & Burke FY. Cognitive function and cerebral blood flow in partial seizures. *Arch. Neurol.*, 1989, 6:964–970.

Jarho L. Korsakoff-like amnesic syndrome in penetrating brain injury. *Acta Neur. Scand.*, 1973, 49:134–137.

Kasteleyn-Nolst Trenité DGA, Siebelink BM, Berends SGC, Van Strien JW & Meinardi H. Lateralized effects of subclinical epileptiform EEG discharges on scholastic performance in children. *Epilepsia*, 1990, 31:740–746.

Kulig BM, Meinarid H & Stores G. (1980). *Epilepsy and behavior '79; proceedings of WOPSASSEPY I.* Lisse: Swets & Zeitlinger.

Ladavas E, Umilta C & Provincialli L. Hemisphere dependent cognitive performance in epileptic patients. *Epilepsia*, 1979, 20:493–502.

The Lancet. Doing better, feeling worse; editorial comments, 1990, 336:1037–1038.

Lezak MD (1976). *Neuropsychological assessment.* New York: Oxford University Press.

Loiseau P, Signoret JL, Strube E, Broustet D, Dartiques JF. Nouveaux procedes d'appreciation des troubles de la memoire chez les epileptiques. *Rev. Neurol.*, 1982, 138:387–400.

Louiseau P, Strube E & Signoret JL. (1987). Memory and epilepsy. In: MR Trimble & EH Reynolds, *Epilepsy, behaviour and cognitive function* (pp. 165–177). Chichester: John Wiley & Sons.

McGlynn SM & Schacter DL. Unawareness of deficits in neuropsychological syndromes. *Journal of Clinical and Experimental Neuropsychology*, 1989(11): 143–205.

McNair DM, Lorr M & Droppleman LF. (1971). *Profile of mood states.* San Diego: Educational and Industrial Testing Service.

Meador KJ, Loring DE, Huh K, Calagher BB & King DW. Comparative cognitive effects of anticonvulsants. *Neurology*, 1990, 40:391–394.

Moerland MC, Aldenkamp AP & Alpherts WCJ. A neuropsychological test battery for the Apple IIE. *Intern. Journ. of Man-Machine Studies*, 1986, 25:453–466.

Moerland MC, Aldenkamp AP & Alpherts WCJ. (1988). Computerized psychological testing in epilepsy. In: FJ Maarse, LJM Mulder, WPB Sjouw & AE Akkerman (eds.), *Computers in psychology: Methods, instrumentation and psychodiagnostics* (pp. 157–164). Swets & Zeitlinger, Lisse/Berwyn (USA).

Neisser, U & Hermann DJ. (1978). An inventory of everyday memory experiences. In: MM Gruneberg, PE Morris & RN Sykes (eds.), *Practical aspects of memory* (pp. 31–51). London: Academic Press.

Ojemann GA & Dodrill CB. Verbal memory deficits after left temporal lobectomy for epilepsy: Mechanisms and intraoperative prediction. *Journ. Neurosurg.*, 1985, 62:101–107.

Ossetin J. (1987). Methods and problems in the assessment of cognitive function in epileptic patients. In: MR Trimble & EH Reynolds (eds.), *Epilepsy, behaviour and cognitive function* (pp. 9–27). Chichester: John Wiley & Sons.

Overweg J, Verhoeff NPLG, van Royen EA, Aldenkamp AP, Verbeeten BWJM & Weinstein H. (1990). *Memory disorders and focus localisation with TC-99M HMPAO SPECT, EE and CT in patients with partial epilepsy* (book of abstracts). Amsterdam: European Nuclear Medicine Congress.

Rodin EA, Schmaltz S & Twitty G. Intellectual functions of patients with childhood-onset epilepsy. *Developmental Medicine & Child Neurology*, 1986, 28:25–33.

Sarason IG, Johnson JH & Siegel JM. Assessing the impact of life changes: Development of the life experiences survey. *Journal of Consulting and Clinical Psychology*, 1978, 932-946.

Schwab RS. Method of measuring consciousness in attacks of petit mal epilepsy. *Arch. Neurol. Psychiatr.*, 1939, 41:215-217.

Scott DF, Moffatt A, Matthews A & Ettlinger G. The effect of epileptic discharges on learning and memory in patients. *Epilepsia*, 1967, 8:188-194.

Shimamura AP & Squire LR. Memory & metamemory: A study of the feeling-of-knowing phenomenon in amnesic patients. *Journal of Experimental Psychology: Learning, Memory and Cognition*, 1986, 12:452-460.

Smith DB, Craft BR, Collins J, Mattson RH & Cramer JA. Behavioural characteristics of epilepsy patients compared with normal controls. *Epilepsia*, 1986, 27: 760-768.

Squire LR, Slater P & Chase PM. Retrograde amnesia: Temporal gradient in very-long-term memory following electroconvulsive therapy. *Science*, 1975, 187: 77-79.

Stores G. Memory impairment in children with epilepsy. *Acta Neur. Scand.*, 1981, 89:21-29.

Sunderland A, Harris JE & Baddeley AD. Do laboratory tests predict everyday memory? A neuropsychological study. *Journal of Verbal Learning and Verbal Behavior*, 1983, 341-357.

Sylfvenius H, Blom S, Nilsson LG, Christianson SA. Observations on verbal, pictorial and stereognostic memory in epileptic patients during intracarotid amytal testing. *Acta Neur. Scand.*, 1984, 99:57-75.

Thompson PJ. (1989). Epilepsy and memory. In: J Manelis, E Bental, JN Loeber & FE Dreifuss (eds.), *Advances in epileptology* (Vol. 17). New York: Raven Press.

Thompson PJ & Huppert F. (1980). Problems in the development of measures to test cognitive performance in adult epileptic patients. In: BM Kulig, H Meinardi & G Stores (eds.), *Epilepsy and behaviour* (pp. 104-111). Amsterdam: Swets & Zeitlinger.

Trimble MR (1987). Anticonvulsant drugs: Mood and cognitive function. In: MR Trimble & EH Reynolds (eds.), *Epilepsy, behaviour and cognitive function* (pp. 135-145). Chichester: John Wiley & Sons.

Trimble MR. Antiepileptic drugs, cognitive function, and behavior in children: Evidence from recent studies. In: AP Aldenkamp & WE Dodson (eds.), Epilepsy and education; cognitive factors in learning behavior. *Epilepsia*, 31(suppl. 4), 1990, pp. S30-S34. New York: Raven Press.

Trimble MR & Reynolds EH. (1987). *Epilepsy, behaviour and cognitive function*. Chichester: John Wiley & Sons.

Trimble MR & Thompson PJ. Anticonvulsant drugs, cognitive function and behavior. *Epilepsia*, 1983, 24 (suppl. 1): pp. S55-S65. New York: Raven Press.

Verhoeff NPLG, Weinstein H, Aldenkamp AP, Overweg J, van Royen EA & Verbeeten BWJ. (In press, 1992). Memory complaints, memory disorders and focus localization in patients with partial epilepsy. *Epilepsia*. New York: Raven Press.

5

Applications of Computerized Cognitive-Motor Measures to the Assessment of Psychoactive Drugs

Michael G. Aman

The Nisonger Center for Mental Retardation and Developmental Disabilities
The Ohio State University

Introduction

This chapter considers the content and function of tests that have been used to assess the effects of psychotropic medications (or to examine various diagnostic groups) in children seen in our laboratory. This discussion includes data on psychometric characteristics of these tests, such as their stability over time, internal consistency, and test–retest reliability. The sensitivity of these tests to various drug treatments and to differences between diagnostic groups is discussed. Then data with intellectually subnormal children provide an indication about how broadly these tests can be applied to children with handicaps, in terms of minimal intellectual maturity and ability required of subjects. Several screens from our laboratory software illustrate the logical structure and flow of the laboratory procedures for the reader. Finally, a number of system advantages and limitations will be described.

Physical Layout of Laboratory

Much of our research has entailed the testing of children with Attention Deficit-Hyperactivity Disorder (ADHD) who have normal IQ, children with epilepsy, and those with the four most common forms of disturbance in the DSM–III diagnostic system, namely conduct, anxiety, attention deficit, and oppositional disorder (Werry et al. 1987). More recently we began to assess children with mental retardation and hyperactivity. Our choice of tests within various batteries depends in part on the specific populations studied.

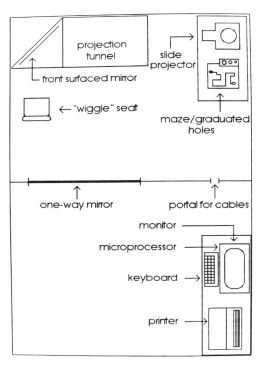

FIGURE 1

Diagram showing the layout of the experimental room and the control room.

Our computerized setup occupies two small rooms, one of which serves as the control room and the other as the examination room. Both rooms are linked by a one-way mirror and by an intercom. There are two additional rooms: one is stocked with prizes to be given to the children after each test session; the other is used for more traditional paper-and-pencil testing. A diagram of the experimental room and the control room appears in Figure 1.

The examination room linked with the computer contains a projection booth that is a tunnel-shaped apparatus with a mirror mounted at a 45-degree angle at one end. All visual (projected) materials are reflected off of this mirror onto response panels positioned in front of the subject's seat. The projection booth is equipped with a hinged metal frame that allows the different panels designed for the various tests to be changed as needed.

Sitting at one end of the projection booth is a table on which two audiovisual carousel slide projectors are mounted. At present, all of our cognitive tests are presented visually by slides or accompanied by tones generated by buzzers in the examination room. The table on which the projectors are mounted also holds a metal slotted maze and a plate with a series of increasingly smaller holes. These items were adapted from Kløve's Motor Steadiness Battery (1963).

In another corner of the room sits a pursuit rotor unit. This is made up of a converted phonograph turntable set to rotate at 16 RPMs. A plate of glass sits on top of the turntable and an opaque mask blocks out all light except for a

1-centimeter circle in the plate. A light assembly mounted on the turntable directs a square centimeter beam of light vertically through the glass; this beam rotates in a circle at 16 RPMs when switched on. The pursuit rotor unit is also equipped with a "wand" that is fitted with a photocell.

Finally, a specially equipped seat is positioned directly before the response panel of the projection tunnel. This seat is modeled after the stabilimetric seat designed by Sprague and Toppe (1966). It is an ordinary chair that has been modified by inserting a fulcrum at the exact centerpoint under the seat cushion, allowing the seat's surface to tilt slightly. A spring at each corner returns the seat to a horizontal position. Microswitches located under each of the four sides of the seat respond to movement. The number of switch closures corresponds roughly to the amount of the subject's wiggle.

All of these units (projection tunnel, slide projectors, motor performance equipment, pursuit rotor console, and wiggle seat) are connected to the computer by a series of cables. The examination room is quiet during test sessions except for the sound of the projector fans, projector advance mechanisms, and auditory signals that are part of the tasks.

Description of the Tests

Most of our studies have been designed to assess the effects of psychotropic drugs. Less often, our investigations have looked at differences between various diagnostic groups. Endeavoring to minimize variance, we hold the order of each test constant because the emphasis has been on the effects of medication or diagnostic group rather than differences between the tests. Our studies often involve repeated testing of the children in order to assess multiple drug conditions. We have therefore developed five parallel versions for most of the tests described here. Our automated tests have been administered usually in the following sequence.

1. Matching Familiar Figures Task

Our task is a modification of that first introduced by Kagan (1965a,b). The child is shown five pictures that are displayed as a standard configuration located at center top of the screen plus four test figures located in a row below the standard. One of the test figures is correct in that it is identical to the standard. The child's task is to identify the matching pictures and depress the corresponding button, which is located directly below the test figures. The position of the correct picture is randomized across trials. Each correct response results in the illumination of a green light on the response panel and the addition of a point to the score displayed on a counter attached to the projection tunnel. If the investigator wishes, the score can be used as an incentive system. Dependent variables include the following: (a) accuracy of responding over

24 trials (12 at a preschool level and 12 at an elementary level of difficulty), (b) mean response time, and (c) mean response speed (defined as the reciprocal of time).

This task is thought to assess a child's visual ability to analyze complex perceptual stimuli. However, the major interest in this task relates to the construct of "reflection-impulsivity" as measured by response time. This is said to indicate a child's tendency to use more or less time to solve problems where a high degree of uncertainty is involved. Aspects of this task predict later reading attainment (Kagan 1965a,b) and are also associated with severe reading disabilities (Aman 1979).

2. Short-Term Memory Task

Originally developed to study models of memory in mentally retarded children (Scott 1971), this task was subsequently adopted to assess drug effects in normal-ability hyperactive children (Sprague & Sleator 1973, 1975, 1977). In our version of the task, a child is shown 3 or 9 pictures extracted from children's books. These pictures are projected either in 1 × 3 or 3 × 3 matrices, onto a display panel for a number of seconds equal to the number of pictures presented. Five seconds after the array of pictures is shown, a single picture is presented in the center of the screen. During half of the trials, this test picture matches one of those in the preceding array; otherwise the test picture differs from those in the previous array. The child is required to decide whether or not the test picture appeared in the previous group and to respond by pressing the "Same" or the "Different" response lever. Each lever is color-coded and identified with the label "Same" or "Different." As in most of the performance tasks, a correct response automatically illuminates the green light and advances the counter. Dependent measures include accuracy, response time, and response speed. This task assesses recognition memory and has been used in the past to study models of memory storage, such as that advocated by Sternberg (1966).

3. Auditory-Visual (A-V) Integration Task

The A-V Integration Task was originally intended to evaluate cross-modal matching by a subject (Birch & Belmont 1964). Operationally, the task usually involves the presentation of a pattern of sounds that are distinguished by long or short intervals between each sound. In our laboratory, the auditory stimuli are tones. Following each sound pattern, a child is shown 4 dot arrangements, one of which matches the sound pattern. The child's task is to locate the correct dot arrangement and to depress the corresponding response button. (We use the same panel for this task for the the Matching Familiar Figures [MFF] task.) Once again, dependent variables include accuracy over 10 trials, response time, and response speed.

A number of studies have shown a consistent relationship between performance on this task and reading ability (Birch & Belmont 1964; Blank & Bridger 1966; Aman 1979). Although originally conceptualized as a test of cross-modal integration, Blank and Bridger demonstrated that this was not the critical function assessed in the task. Rather, the child's ability to translate stimuli from a temporal to a spatial dimension appears to be at issue.

4. Memory Distraction Task

We developed this task anew because of our interest in the triad of inattention, impulsivity, and distractability in children with ADHD; specifically, this task is intended to assess proneness to distraction (Aman et al. 1987a). Functionally, the task involves the presentation of triangular and square patterns similar to the block design subscales of the Wechsler IQ tests. After each block pattern is presented, it is followed 3 s later by 4 block patterns. The child's task is to locate the identical pattern among the test stimuli and to depress the corresponding response button. The critical part of this task entails the introduction of distracting stimuli (salient pictures taken from comic and story books) around the block patterns. Performance is assessed for 16 trials each under both distracting and nondistracting conditions. Accuracy, response time, and response speed are analyzed separately for the two conditions.

5. Delayed Matching-to-Sample (MTS) Task

This task has been used extensively with laboratory animals, such as pigeons, to assess drug effects on memory performance (Cumming & Berryman 1965). Recently, we adapted it for use in evaluating pharmacotherapy in children with mental retardation (Aman et al. 1991b). Operationally, the task requires the child to observe a panel having four windows—one at center top and three positioned below. Three colors are projected onto the windows: yellow, blue, and red. First, a color is projected onto the top window and this remains illuminated until the child presses the aperture (observing response). One second later, all three colors appear on the bottom windows, and the child is required to press the window with the matching color. Correct responses result in a green light being illuminated on the panel for 1 s.

This task is titrated in the sense that better performance results in a longer delay between the original stimulus and the test colors. Each time the child obtains three consecutive correct responses, a second is added to the delay between original and test stimuli. Each incorrect response results in a reduction to the delay interval by 1 s, with the provision that the interval never shrinks to less than 1 s. Dependent variables include accuracy, longest delay achieved, mean response time, and mean response speed. We find this to be a very useful task with mentally retarded children, as many of these subjects (even those with quite low IQs) can perform this task successfully.

6. Continuous Performance Task (CPT)

This task (and variations thereof) is probably the single most commonly used performance measure in pediatric psychopharmacology (Aman 1978). The task first became popular in research with hyperactive children following a study by Sykes and colleagues (1971) who showed that hyperactive children performed at a deficit that improved with psychostimulant medication. Most workers regard the CPT as a test of sustained attention.

In its simplest format, the task involves the serial presentation of visual or auditory stimuli, one of which is designated as the target stimulus. The subject is required to respond when the target appears and to refrain from responding when the alternative simuli appear. In a more complex version, the subject is instructed to respond to the target if it is preceded by another specific stimulus. In the Sykes et al. study (1971), the target was the letter X which was to be responded to only if preceded by an A.

In our studies we employ the simpler version of the CPT because ours appears to be purer measure of attention. In other words, the child does not need to remember whether the letter A appeared on the previous trial. Depending on the experimental question, we have worked with four versions of the task using the following stimuli: (a) 10 characters from the alphabet, with X designated as the target, and with a constant interstimulus interval; (b) 4 stimuli from the Illinois Test of Psycholinguistic Abilities, which were very similar in appearance, with 1 character designated as the target; (c) 2 letters (X and O), presented on a one-plane readout for very brief durations (0.3s), with variable interstimulus intervals (3–5 s), and with the X designated as the target; and (d) pictures of the fairytale character, Snow White, and a witch shown for intervals of 2 s each and with a constant intersimulus interval of 1 s. In contrast to the other tests, no feedback is given to the subject (e.g., via green lights) regarding the accuracy of his or her responding during this task. Dependent variables include errors of omission (failures to detect the target), errors of commission (incorrect detections), mean response time, and mean response speed. Version (c) (above) is most suitable for studies in children of normal ability. Version (d) produces favorable results in children with mental retardation.

7. Seat Activity

Most of our studies involve hyperactive children; therefore, the amount of activity during laboratory testing is relevant. During all of the tests described above, seat movement is recorded using the special wiggle seat described above. Because the response interval is variable for many of these tasks, contingent on subject response time, the computer is programmed to calculate the number of seat wiggles divided by the time for each trial. Also, subjects often tend to lean forward in the activity seat when responding appropriately during the CPT. The computer has therefore been programmed to ignore seat activity that occurs during trials in which the target is presented. These refinements tend to strengthen the likelihood of observing significant changes due to experimental manipulations. The dependent measures typically collected with the activity seat include (a) activity only during the constant portions of each task, and (b) total time-corrected activity for the entire task, including the variable response intervals.

8. Graduated Holes Task

As noted earlier, this has been adapted from Kløve's Motor Steadiness Battery (1963). The child is required to hold a stylus, for 10 s each in five holes, while trying not to make contact with the sides. This is done with each hand for the five largest holes, which are graduated from large to small. The number of contacts and the time of contact are automatically recorded for each hand separately and totaled over both hands. The task probably measures a composite of static tremor and sustained attention.

9. Maze Task

In this task a child is required to run a stylus through a metal maze while avoiding contact with the sides. The base of the maze is made of glass. Any contact between the stylus and the sides of the maze closes an electrical circuit and is recorded as an error measure. Dependent variables include contact time, number of contacts, and the ratio of error time to total travel time. This test is presumed to assess dynamic tremor and eye–hand coordination.

10. Pursuit Rotor Task

As noted earlier, this test uses a modified phonograph turntable with a mechanism that directs a square beam vertically through a plate of glass as it rotates at 16 RPMs. We regard this primarily as a test of eye–hand coordination, although attention span may also be assessed to some degree. A child's task is to track the light beam using a wand fitted with a photocell. Three trials of 10 s each are performed with each hand. The role of the computer in this task is to regulate the duration of each trial and to time the amount of contact for each hand.

Psychometric Characteristics

In this section we discuss the internal consistency, temporal stability, and reliability of some of our tests. In addition, we present data on the sensitivity of these measures to drug and subject variables and the suitability of certain tests for children with subaverage intelligence.

TABLE 1

Alpha Coefficients for Performance Tests Administered Two Years Apart

Test	Initial Alpha	Follow-up Alpha
Matching Familiar Figures		
Accuracy (%)	.557	.399
Response Time (sec)	.900	.907
Auditory-Visual Integration		
Accuracy (%)	.695	.689
Response Speed (1/sec)	.860	.556
Short-Term Memory		
Accuracy (%)	.531	.373
Response Speed (1/sec)	.920	.897
Continuous Performance Task		
Omission Errors (%)	.294	.743
Response Time (sec)	.894	.962
Seat Movement		
Matching Familiar Figures	.870	.909
Auditory-Visual Integration	.925	.827

Note: Data are reproduced by permission from Aman and Mayhew (1980).

Internal Consistency

Aman and Mayhew (1980) assessed the internal consistency (or the extent to which the test items assessed the same attribute) of several of these tests in 28 children with severe reading disabilities. The children were assessed at initial contact, when their mean age was 9.9 years, and at follow-up 2 years later. Alpha coefficients were calculated for each of the dependent variables, both on initial assessment and at the time of follow-up.

In general, the alpha coefficients ranged from quite modest (e.g., 0.294 for omission errors on the CPT at initial testing) to very high (e.g., 0.962 for response time on the CPT at follow-up). The suitability of these tasks varies in part with age, with accuracy-type variables often showing less internal consistency with greater age (i.e., at the time of follow-up). Also it is interesting to note that measures of response time are very robust with this particular statistic. These data provide limited support for the potential reliability of these tests, but it must be remembered that the data are derived from only one sample of children who had severe reading disorders.

Stability and Test-Retest Reliability

Another issue relates to the amount of change that occurs over successive test sessions with the various tasks. In our drug studies, we allow for one or two extra sessions before starting the actual experimental sessions because performance tends to stabilize after one practice or "familiarization" session. Performance tasks that entail the development of skills or strategies typically show a practice effect manifested by improvement from the first to second session. On the other hand, performance on monotonous tasks frequently deteriorates, indicating boredom. Thereafter, performance seems to stabilize greatly. In all of our drug studies, we counterbalance drug treatment sequences to eliminate the effect of any residual practice effects.

The next data are from three studies of children with epilepsy taking phenytoin, carbamazepine, or sodium valproate monotherapy (Aman et al. 1987b, 1990b, 1991c). The design for all three studies called for a familiarization session (test 1), assessment midmorning following usual dosing, and assessment midmorning with the morning medication delayed until after testing. These two conditions (medication before testing and medication delayed until after testing) were assessed during sessions 2 and 3 and comprised the critical comparison. The two conditions (i.e., medication before testing; medication delayed) were counterbalanced across sessions 2 and 3 and across all three drugs, so that the net effect on average should have balanced out to no change across the entire group. Thus, we also have an opportunity to examine the stability of performance with these tests, although we should bear in mind that any medication effects may influence the upper limits of stability and reliability.

The first 54 participants of the three drug studies were entered into this comparison. Their ages ranged from 4.2 years to 14 years, with a mean of 9.45 years. Twenty-three of the subjects (43%) were boys, and 31 were girls. Twenty-six subjects were taking phenytoin monotherapy, 15 carbamazepine monotherapy, and 13 sodium valproate monotherapy.

The mean scores for performance tests across sessions are shown in Table 2. In general there is a steep rise in performance, from session 1 to session 2, on tasks involving skill acquisition. Performance usually levels off thereafter. However, for tests involving boredom, such as the CPT, there is some indication of continued worsening across sessions. With a few exceptions, performance tends to approach a plateau after a single familiarization session.

To test the reliability of performance across sessions, we correlated performance between each possible pairwise combination of sessions. This relates only to the lower limits of test–retest reliability because some drug effects (although generally modest in impact) were presumably operative across these sessions. The Pearson correlations range from essentially zero to very high (.96) (Table 3). Because of the marked learning that takes place between the first and the second session, we predicted that the correlations would be highest between sessions 2 and 3. In fact, the mean correlation for pairwise comparisons of sessions 1 to 3 were .65, .60, and .71, with highest reliability between sessions 2 and 3. Inspection of the data from the right-most column of Table 3 indicates that reliability levels are highest for motor performance measures, which had

TABLE 2

Stability of Performance on Cognitive-Motor Tasks Over Three Sessions

	Mean Scores		
Testing Tasks	Session 1	Session 2	Session 3
Matching Familiar Figures (MFF)			
Accuracy (%)	75.42	80.49	81.11
Time (sec)	9.73	8.82	9.28
Auditory-Visual (A-V) Integration			
Accuracy (%)	71.14	76.25	81.00
Time (sec)	5.43	4.44	4.82
Short-Term Memory (STM)			
Accuracy (%)	80.17	84.67	81.58
Time (sec)	2.81	2.66	2.66
Continuous Performance Task (CPT)			
Omissions	1.79	2.40	3.48
Commissions	1.95	1.42	1.92
Time	37.51	42.06	44.96
Seat Movement			
MFF	12.91	20.30	21.03
A-V Integration	8.44	12.73	11.44
STM	18.51	39.72	46.22
CPT	25.12	44.77	53.37
Maze			
Contact Time	6.68	6.21	6.10
Errors	42.23	39.85	39.02
Ratio	0.144	0.141	0.150
Graduated Holes			
Contact Time	20.50	21.36	20.92
Number of Errors	144.08	139.17	143.38
Pursuit Rotor			
Contact Time	18.52	26.81	28.77

Notes: Data taken from Aman et al. (1987b, 1990, 1991c). Subjects were children with epilepsy whose time of medication was modified during session 2 or session 3. Changes in medication time were balanced across sessions 2 and 3 (see text).

correlation coefficients in the .80 and .90 range. Reliability was quite modest for seat movement and Short-Term Memory performance, whereas it was moderately high for the MFF, Auditory-Visual Integration, and Continuous Performance tasks. However, we again emphasize that these may be low estimates of true reliability levels for these tests because they are from sessions in which a drug manipulation took place. Also, tests were of very brief duration: seldom did they last longer than 10 minutes.

TABLE 3

Reliability of Performance on Cognitive-Motor Tasks Over Three Sessions

Testing Tasks	Reliability Levels		
	Sessions 1 & 2	Sessions 1 & 3	Sessions 2 & 3
Matching Familiar Figures (MFF)			
Accuracy (%)	.78	.73	.78
Time (sec)	.81	.56	.74
Auditory-Visual (A-V) Integration			
Accuracy (%)	.71	.46	.68
Time (sec)	.75	.83	.66
Short-Term Memory (STM)			
Accuracy (%)	.49	.39	.42
Time (sec)	.51	.43	.75
Continuous Performance Task (CPT)			
Omissions	.75	.83	.81
Commissions	.43	.34	.87
Time	.63	.76	.80
Seat Movement			
MFF	.49	.14	.31
A-V Integration	.36	.53	.55
STM	.07	.26	.53
CPT	.46	.16	.42
Maze			
Contact Time	.93	.96	.93
Number Errors	.75	.86	.89
Ratio	.83	.89	.71
Graduated Holes			
Contact Time	.85	.85	.94
Number of Errors	.79	.62	.80
Pursuit Rotor			
Contact Time	.89	.72	.89
Column Means	.65	.60	.71

Notes: Data taken from Aman et al. (1987b, 1990, 1991c). Subjects were children with epilepsy whose time of medication was modified during session 2 or session 3. Changes in medication time were balanced across sessions 2 and 3 (see text).

Sensitivity of the Cognitive-Motor Battery

A major question regarding any test battery relates to its practical utility: How sensitive is the test to treatment effects and to relevant differences between subject groups? In an attempt to examine this issue, 13 studies that used automated tests in our laboratories were individually tabulated. Each of

TABLE 4

Sensitivity of Cognitive-Motor Tests to Experimental Conditions

Authors	Matching Familiar Figures — Acc.	Matching Familiar Figures — Time	Auditory-Visual Integration — Acc.	Auditory-Visual Integration — Time	Short-Term Memory — Acc.	Short-Term Memory — Time	Continuous Performance — Om.	Continuous Performance — Comm.	Continuous Performance — Time	Seat Movement — MFF	Seat Movement — A-V	Seat Movement — STM	Seat Movement — CPT	Maze Task — Error Time	Maze Task — Errors	Maze Task — Ratio	Graduated Holes — Error Time	Graduated Holes — Errors	Pursuit Rotor — Time of Contact
Aman & Sprague (1974)					NS	NS	S	S	NS			S	NS						
Werry & Aman (1975)		NS			S	NS	S	S	†			NS	NS						
Aman (1979) Group	S		S	S			S	S	S		NS	S	S					NS	
Werry, Aman & Diamond (1980)		NS	NS	NS	NS	NS	S	NS	NS			S	S	NS	NS	S	NS	S	
Aman & Werry (1982)	NS	NS	NS	NS	NS	NS	S	NS	S		NS	S	S	NS	NS		S	S	
Werry & Aman (1984) Drug					†	†	S	S	NS	S		S	S				†	S	
Werry & Aman (1984) Group					NS	S	S	NS	NS			NS	NS				S	S	
Aman, Vamos & Werry (1984)	NS	NS								NS		NS	S						
Aman, Mitchell & Turbott (1987a)	NS	NS			S	NS	S	NS	NS	NS	NS	NS	NS	NS	NS	S	NS	NS	
Aman, Werry, Paxton & Turbott (1987b) Group	NS	NS	NS	S	NS	S	S	S	NS	NS	NS	†	NS	NS	NS	S	NS	NS	†
Aman, Werry, Paxton & Turbott (1987b) Dose	NS	NS	S	S	NS	NS				S	NS	NS	NS	NS	S	NS	NS	NS	
Aman, Werry, Paxton, Turbott & Stewart (1990)	NS	S	NS	S	NS	S	NS	S	NS	NS	NS	S	S	NS	NS	†	NS	S	NS
Aman & Turbott (1991)	S	S			NS	S	S	S	NS	S		S	S	NS	NS	NS	S	S	S
Aman, Marks, Turbott, Wilsher & Merry (1991b)	NS	NS			NS	†	S	NS	NS	NS		NS	NS				†	NS	
Werry, Elkind & Reeves (1987) Group	S	NS					NS	NS	†	NS		NS	NS	S	S	S	S	NS	
Totals																			
Not Significant	6	7	3	1	8	6	5	6	9	5	5	6	7	7	7	2	5	6	1
Marginal †		2			1	2		2	2		0	1				1			1
Significant	3	2	2	4	2	3	8	7	2	3	0	5	5	2	2	2	4	4	1
Efficiency	33	22	40	80	20	33	62	54	18	38	0	45	42	22	22	50	44	40	50

KEY: Acc. = accuracy, Om. = omission errors, Comm. = commission errors, MFF = matching familiar figures, STM = short-term memory, CPT = continuous performance test, A.-V = auditory-visual integration, NS = not significant, † = marginal, S = significant, Efficiency = percentage of S + NS comparisons in which a given variable was statistically significant.

the tasks described above was examined to see if the resulting dependent variables discriminated between the various experimental conditions. The variable was tagged with an *S* if the finding was statistically significant (i.e., *p*, < .05, two-tailed), with an *NS* if the comparison was not significant, and a dagger (†) if the outcome was marginal (i.e., .05 < *p* < .10). Then each dependent variable was classified in terms of the number of times it was found to be a significant discriminator of the experimental manipulation (see Table 4).

We arbitrarily classified each variable as having low (0–29%), below average (30–39%), above average (40–49%), and very high (50%+) sensitivity based on the rate of significant findings for that variable. As can be seen from Table 4, MFF time, short-term memory (STM) accuracy, CPT time, A-V Integration seat movement, and Maze error time and number of errors all tended to be relatively insensitive measures. MFF accuracy, STM time, and MFF seat movement were classed as having below-average sensitivity. A-V Integration accuracy, seat movement on both the STM and CPT tasks, and Graduated Holes error time and number of errors were relatively sensitive ("above average") to the presence of experimental variables. Finally A-V Integration response time, CPT omission and commission errors, and Maze ratio scores were all very robust indicators ("very high" sensitivity) of treatment effectiveness or diagnostic differences. This is interesting, as the CPT has long been regarded as one of the most frequently used and highly sensitive tasks in drug studies with children (Aman 1978). However, these findings suggest that both the A-V Integration task and the Maze task may warrant more use in these types of studies.

Computer Testing in Children with Subaverage IQs

We recently completed a drug study in 30 children having subaverage IQs and hyperactivity or a conduct disorder (Aman et al. 1991b). Their ages ranged from 4.1 to 16.5 years (Mean [*M*] = 10.0), and their IQs ranged from untestable to 90 (*M* = 52.3). The study was carried out in two localities in Auckland, New Zealand, but only one of these had the automated assessment laboratory. Children seen at the second location (i.e., the one without the cognitive-motor tests) were tested solely on clinical response measures. We tended to arrange appointments partly based on convenience for the families concerned and partly based on our impression of whether a given child could perform the tests. The question of interest here is how well these exceptional children could perform the tests.

The numbers of children able to carry out the tests are presented in Figure 2 and Figure 3. In Figure 2, successful performance is portrayed as a function of IQ level. Only 2 of 12 subjects (17%) with IQs below 40 could comply with the test procedures. However, most of those with IQs greater than 40 could provide meaningful data with these tests. In Figure 3, ability to perform is presented

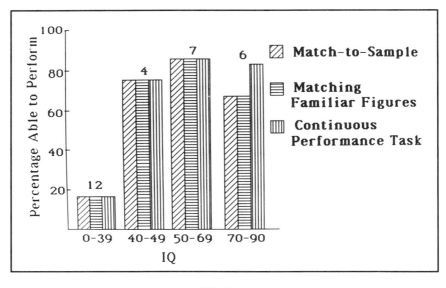

FIGURE 2

Ability to perform selected cognitive tests as a function of IQ level. Numbers above bars indicate numbers of subjects falling within that IQ range. Data are abstracted from Aman et al. (1991b).

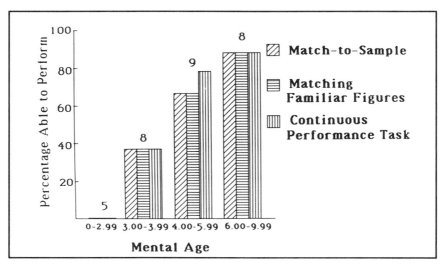

FIGURE 3

Ability to perform selected cognitive tests as a function of Mental Age (MA) are assessed on the Stanford–Binet Intelligence Scale (3d ed.). Numbers above bars signify the numbers of subjects falling within that MA range. Data are abstracted from Aman et al. (1991b).

as a function of mental age (MA). Nearly half of those with an MA between 3.00 and 3.99 years could carry out the test procedures. Between 67% and 88% of those with MAs above 4.00 years could conduct the tests. As noted above, not all of the children actually attempted to do these tests, so that these figures may underestimate the number of children with low IQs who can perform such tasks.

At the time of this writing we are in the process of completing another study with 30 children selected for mental retardation with severe hyperactivity (Aman et al. 1991a). The children range in age from 5 to 13 years ($M = 8.8$), and IQs extend from unmeasurable to 78 ($M = 50.1$). The data on their ability to comply with computer test procedures are portrayed in Figure 4 and Figure 5. In this study, only a minority of children having IQs between 40 and 49 could successfully meet test requirements. However, all of those with IQs greater than 49 could do the tests (Figure 4). Figure 5 depicts the children's ability to comply with testing requirements as a function of their MA equivalents on the Stanford–Binet Intelligence Test (4th ed.). Interestingly, by the time children acquired an MA equivalent of 3.00 years, the majority were able to perform the tests. Conversely, only a minority of youngsters with MA equivalents below 3.00 years could comply.

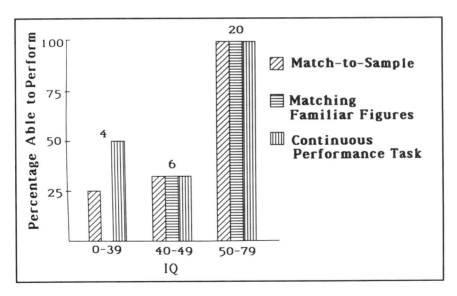

FIGURE 4

Ability to perform selected cognitive tests as a function of IQ level. Numbers above bars indicate the numbers of subjects falling within that IQ range. Data are abstracted from Aman et al. (1991a).

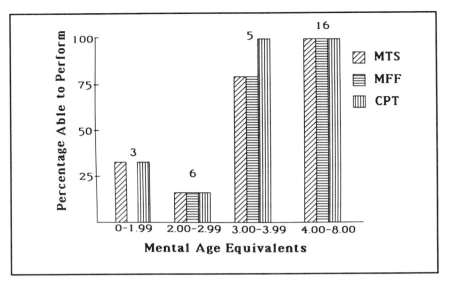

FIGURE 5

Ability to perform selected cognitive tests as a function of Mental Age (MA) equivalents on the Stanford–Binet Intelligence Scale (4th ed.). Numbers above bars indicate the numbers of subjects falling within that MA range. Data are abstracted from Aman et al. (1991a).

As illustrated in figures 2 to 5, the numbers of children within each of the IQ and MA ranges were very small. Notwithstanding, these results suggest that it is possible to derive meaningful cognitive data with relatively little pretraining from a large proportion of handicapped children. This was true despite the presence of severe hyperactivity or other behavior disorders. Success falls off quite dramatically below an MA of 3.00 years and below an IQ of roughly 40 to 50. Although it was not feasible to do so in these studies, greater success could be achieved with additional training of the children using shaping and reinforcement procedures.

Organization of Laboratory Tests

We will now describe the way we structure our software by the use of screens that guide the user through the test process. The screens that appear are similar regardless of the task. All tasks follow a similar logic. The first screen (Figure 6) automatically appears when the self-booting program is initiated and presents two principal options. The first will result in the main menu of tasks appearing on the monitor. The second option *T* results in a test program for assessing the electric circuitry of the apparatus. This has been invaluable for initial wiring of

```
┌─────────────────────────────────────────┐
│            Welcome  to                  │
│                                         │
│  The  Psychomotor  Test  Laboratory     │
│     for   Assessing   Children          │
│                                         │
│                                         │
│          Date:    3/09/1991             │
│          Time:  10:44:45                │
│                                         │
│                                         │
│                                         │
│ Press  <Enter> to main menu             │
│        <Esc> to Disk Operating System   │
│        <S> to set the time              │
│        <T> to check the circuits        │
└─────────────────────────────────────────┘
```

FIGURE 6

"Welcome" screen obtained upon initiating computer test system. Functions are activated by depressing the "Enter," "Esc," "S," or "T" keys on the keyboard.

```
┌─────────────────────────────────────────┐
│                                         │
│            TEST CIRCUITS                │
│                                         │
│                                         │
│      INPUT          OUTPUT              │
│    ┌──────────┬──────────┐              │
│    │   PA1    │   PB1    │              │
│    │   PA2    │   PB2    │              │
│    │   PA3    │   PB3    │              │
│    │   PA4    │   PB4    │              │
│    │   PA5    │   PB5    │              │
│    │   PA6    │   PB6    │              │
│    │   PA7    │   PB7    │              │
│    │   PA8    │   PB8    │              │
│    └──────────┴──────────┘              │
│                                         │
│                                         │
│   PRESS 1,2,3,4,5,6,7,8 for output      │
│         testing                         │
│                                         │
│   PRESS <Q> to stop testing             │
│                                         │
└─────────────────────────────────────────┘
```

FIGURE 7

Display for the Test program. Depressing numeric keys 1 through 8 activates each of the respective output circuits. Activation of input circuits results in illumination of the respective input cell and a unique auditory tone for each input channel.

the system and for troubleshooting when hardware faults occur (see Figure 7). The Test program allows the user to activate each of 8 output channels simply by depressing digits 1 to 8 on the keyboard. The user can also test all input channels in similar fashion. Whenever an input signal is simulated, the computer sounds a unique tone and illuminates the relevant numeric cell on the monitor. In this way we can check for hardware problems, such as broken connections or severed wires.

```
┌─────────────────────────────────────────────┐
│              Behavioral   Tests               │
├─────────────────────────────────────────────┤
│                                               │
│   1. Delayed  Matching-To-Sample  Task        │
│   2. Matching Familiar Figures Task           │
│   3. Short term Memory Task                    │
│   4. Continuous Performance Task (EASY)        │
│   5. Continuous Performance Task (HARD)        │
│   6. Memory  Distraction  Task                 │
│   7. Maze Task                                 │
│   8. Graduated  Holes  Task                    │
│   9. Auditory-Visual  Integration  Task        │
│  10. Pursuit  Rotor  Task                      │
│  11. Quit                                      │
│                                               │
├─────────────────────────────────────────────┤
│     move  cursor          <ENTER> select      │
└─────────────────────────────────────────────┘
```

FIGURE 8

Main menu for the test battery. Tests are chosen by highlighting the desired selection with the cursor and depressing the Enter key.

```
┌─────────────────────────────────────────┐
│                                          │
│      Delayed Matching-to-                │
│         Sample  Task                     │
│                                          │
├─────────────────────────────────────────┤
│                                          │
│   1. Begin  Task                         │
│   2. Inquire  about  Previous            │
│      Data                                │
│   3. Input  or  Modify  Trial            │
│      Sequence                            │
│   4. Quit                                │
│                                          │
├──────────────────────┬──────────────────┤
│ move    cursor       │ <ENTER> select    │
└──────────────────────┴──────────────────┘
```

FIGURE 9

Screen for the Matching-to-Sample task. The user selects the appropriate function by highlighting that choice and depressing the Enter key.

The next screen (Figure 8) shows the menu of tests. The user indicates his or her choice by moving the cursor (which results in a highlighting of the line of print) using the up (↑) or the down (↓) key and depressing Enter. (For purposes of illustration, we will show the various menus for the Matching-to-Sample task.)

Once the task is selected, a new screen appears (Figure 9) providing the operator four choices: Begin Task, Inquire about Previous Data, Input or Modify Trial Sequence, and Quit. Highlighting the first choice results in a screen requesting subject and study identification information (Figure 10). For the top half of this screen, the user simply enters the relevant information regarding the subject, date, study, and so forth. Because this information is automatically carried forward to all subsequent tasks it does not need to be entered more than once a day. The bottom half of this screen defaults to a set of predetermined parameters for each task. The operator can endorse these default parameters by depressing Enter, or can modify any or all of them. The default parameters suffice for the vast majority of subjects tested and studied in our laboratory. However, we can change these if appropriate (e.g., if the subjects are normal adults).

Request and Print out	
(a) Subject's name: Doe, John	
(b) Date(month/day/year): 3/08/91	
(c) Session: test	
(d) Study name: Fenfluramine	

Did you input the data completely (Y/N)?

(Press ENTER for default value)

Initial delay = 1.0 (sec).
Delay increase = 1.0 (sec).
Delay decrease = 1.0 (sec).
Counter_cycle = 3.0 (# consecutive correct responses needed before increase occurs)
Number of trials: 36

Are the parameters ok (Y/N)?

FIGURE 10

Screen to initiate Matching-to-Sample task. The user enters relevant identification data in top half. Typically the operator simply endorses the preestablished task parameters (by entering Y), although these can be overridden if appropriate.

Delayed   Matching-to-Sample

Trial No.	Corr.	Delay	Resp. Win.	Resp. Time	Resp. Speed	NSM	TSM	Total Time
1	Yes	1.00	2	1.05	.952	2	4	6.04
2	Yes	1.00	1	.94	1.064	4	4	5.93
3	Yes	1.00	2	.72	1.389	0	6	8.68
4	No	2.00	3	.83	1.205	9	1 3	6.60
.								
.								
.								
3 6								

Intertrial interval   Sample on   Delay Buzzer Test stimuli Print out

FIGURE 11

Screen showing the subject's performance as it unfolds. Recurring phases of the task are shown at the very bottom of the figure. During testing, the appropriate phase is highlighted on the monitor and accompanied by a unique tone. In this way, the examiner can monitor the routine "pulse" of each test session.

User's   break

1. Finish current trial then Delay
2. Delay the Task
3. End test and save results
4. End test and abandon results
5. Finish current trial then End
6. Continue the test at specified trial
7. Continue the test
Esc = Go back to the test immediately

FIGURE 12

Screen showing user options when the "panic switch" is depressed. By highlighting the appropriate option and depressing the Enter key the operator can deal appropriately with any eventuality during a test session.

If the test goes smoothly, the user has to take no further action. All information is presented on the monitor as the test unfolds, and it is printed out trial by trial. The monitor display (depicted in Figure 11) enables the examiner to observe any difficulties, such as the development of response sets, unusually lengthy or brief response times, and so forth. Occasionally some unforeseen event (such as the subject's need to take a toilet break) necessitates interrupting the test procedure. This is done by depressing the Escape key (known affectionately in our laboratory as the "panic button"), which results in options for stopping and/or resuming the test (see Figure 12). Most often the examiner opts simply to delay and then to resume the test once the difficulty is resolved. However, if continuity is important, the examiner can return to an earlier stage of the test and repeat several trials before resuming the final stages of the test (see option 6 of Figure 12).

Finally, on completion of the task, the results are both printed automatically and saved on a floppy disk. The printout contains a variety of summary statistics including (a) accuracy of responding, (b) mean response time, (c) mean response speed, (d) longest delay achieved, (e) mean delay over the full test, (f) the number of "net" seat movements (i.e., for those portions of the test that are held constant), and (g) number of seat movements per second (see Figure 13). The total number of trials successfully completed and the number of times each type of response is made are also reported.

Delayed Matching-to-Sample		
(a) Subject ID:		
(1) Name:	Doe, John	
(2) Date:	3/08/91	
(3) Session #:	I	
(4) Name of study:	fenfluramine	
(b) Summary data (for 36 trials) Form No. 1		
(1) Mean accuracy:		83.33%
(2) Mean response time		1.198 (sec)
(3) Mean response speed		1.012
(4) Longest delay achieved		6.00 (sec)
(5) Mean delay		3.47 (sec)
(6) Net set movements:		23
(7) Total seat movements/time:		0.17
Reference data:		
(1) No. times correct:	30	
(2) Responses left:	11	right: 12
center:	13	no response: 0
(3) Total seat movements:	61	
(4) Total time:	350.10 (sec)	

FIGURE 13

Printout of summary data for the Matching-to-Sample task.

Other than control of the test procedures, there are two additional important functions offered under the options for each task. The first concerns the creation of trial sequences (i.e., the position of correct responses) for new or parallel forms of the task. This is achieved simply by highlighting the correct position (left, center, right) on the monitor using the arrow keys and the Enter key (see Figure 14 and Figure 15).

The other imortant function is the Inquiry system. This enables the examiner the option to review, edit, or delete (erase) results that were recorded (saved) on the floppy disk (see Figure 16 and Figure 17). This is a necessary option if the information saved on disk is wrong as might occur when a slide jams during testing causing the computer software to score a response incorrectly as an error. Using the edit function, the examiner may override the computer's scoring by deleting the incorrect trial. Similarly, old or unwanted records may be deleted easily.

Delayed Matching-to-
Sample Task
input or change correct trial
sequence

1. Create new trial sequence
   file
2. Modify trial sequence file
3. Quit

move cursor | <ENTER> select

Delayed Matching-to-Sample Task
Modify correct trial sequence - Form 1

1	Left	Center	Right
2	Left	Center	Right
3	Left	Center	Right
4	Left	Center	Right
5	Left	Center	Right
6	Left	Center	Right
7	Left	Center	Right
8	Left	Center	Right
9	Left	Center	Right
10	Left	Center	Right
11	Left	Center	Right
12	Left	Center	Right
13	Left	Center	Right

Move arrow to select correct resp.
Press <Enter> to end the input

Page Up: Previous Page
Page Down: Next Page

F1
Help

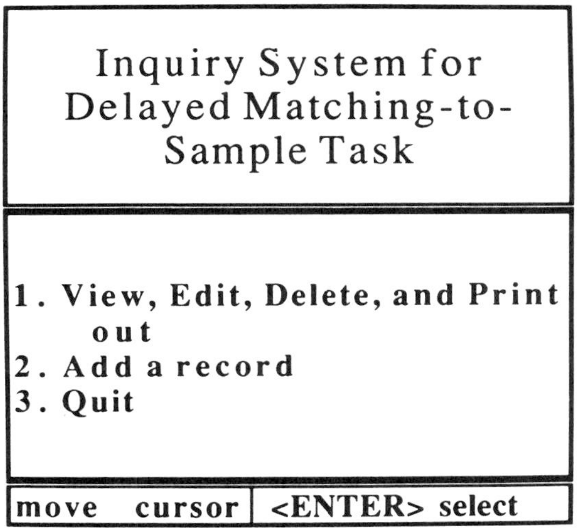

FIGURE 16

Screen for branching to edit (Inquiry) system.

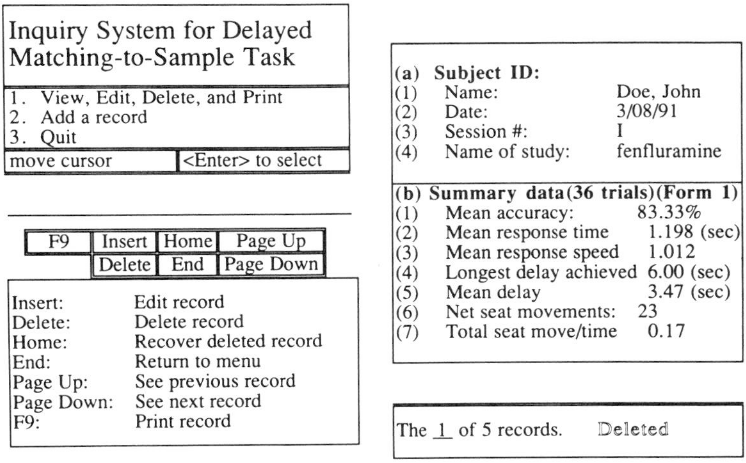

FIGURE 17

Screen for altering records already stored on floppy disk.

Some Strengths and Weaknesses of the Current System

Strengths

No attempt will be made here to enumerate the many advantages realized by employing automated control of experimental procedures, as these have been well reviewed previously (e.g., Cull & Trimble 1987). Instead, we shall identify the major advantages as they impact our specific area of research.

Objectivity. It seems almost trite to cite this feature because it has been singled out by so many other investigators. Nevertheless, the enhanced objectivity provided by computer assessments takes on special importance where human bias about what ought to occur comes into play. In our studies, we often have strong preconceptions of what should transpire. Automated procedures are good antidotes to this type of bias.

Flexibility. Our performance tests have been enormously versatile regardless of subject characteristics, such as age, first language spoken by the child, and IQ differences. Generally speaking, the tasks can be readily adapted for different ability levels by changing certain task parameters, such as the number of stimuli to be processed or the durations of stimuli. The tasks are culture-fair and require minimal formal education for a child to comply. The result is that most of the tests making up this battery can be mastered by the large majority of children likely to be seen in many clinics or research centers.

Nonthreatening Character. Our stimuli do not resemble the paper-and-pencil tests on which many exceptional children have experienced failure because the stimuli here are largely audio tones and photographic images. Most of our subjects actually enjoy the assessment process. This can become a critical factor in the success or failure of any study. Most of our drug studies have within-subject, crossover designs requiring repeated testing. The allegiance of the children themselves is vital to the success of these investigations.

Weaknesses

Over the years, various limitations with our automated system have become apparent. These are nuisances rather than serious handicaps. All of these problems relate in one way or another to the presentation of visual stimuli.

Problems with Photographic Slides. Although slides provide a versatile way of capturing visual material, the duplication process is very labor-intensive. It is also an exacting process. Unless great care is taken to ensure uniform techniques (such as use of a precise template, constant positioning of camera and stimuli, and uniform light intensity) imperfections in the stimuli result. Further, it can be challenging to squeeze all of the necessary detail onto a 35 mm slide format. In a similar vein, very small errors in placement of the transparency within the slide mount can result in large discrepancies in positioning the projected images. These problems pose the single biggest limitation with our current system.

Delays Within the Projectors. Most Kodak Audiovisual carousel projectors require about 1 s to advance. This of course limits how fast stimuli can be presented. Although this has not affected our selection of tests to date, it could do so in the future.

Coordination of Computer and Slide Projector. Correct computer control of the slide projector assumes that both are synchronized. Occasionally the alignment between the computer and slide projector can be lost, as when a subject requires extra warm-up trials before actually starting a test (requiring manual repositioning of the slide tray), or when a test session is interrupted because of a toilet break. If the expected number of trials is altered, then the operator needs to calculate the correct position on the slide tray. Insofar as this coordination is not automated, a potential for error exists.

Conclusions

The automation of a variety of cognitive-motor tests for use in monitoring psychoactive drugs in children has proven to be fairly straightforward. Computerized testing can be highly efficient because the software can automatically calculate and store relevant summary statistics for each subject. Although the data are limited, the psychometric characteristics of these tasks are acceptable to good, especially considering the brief duration of most of these tasks. Many of the tasks have average to very good sensitivity to treatment effects, and the tests are remarkably flexible. Indeed many have even been used successfully with children who have hyperactivity and/or mental retardation. We have developed a software system that is very user-friendly and yet responsive to the complications that occur when testing exceptional children. The major weakness with our current system involves the presentation of visual stimuli. However, this shortcoming is greatly outweighed by its advantages, which include enhanced objectivity, flexibility, and attractiveness to children.

As noted by others, technology has brought us to a point where the major limitation on what can be tested by computers is imposed by our imagination (or lack of imagination). Sophisticated methods are now available both for presenting complex stimuli and for inputting a multitude of subject responses, making it possible to consider computer assessments for virtually any type of cognitive or motor function one wishes to test.

Acknowledgments

Much of the work reported in this chapter was done in collaboration with John S. Werry, M.D., and Robert L. Sprague, Ph.D. The author wishes to note their contributions both to the research designs and development of procedures discussed here. The author is grateful to Deb McGhee who prepared many of the figures presented here.

The research discussed was supported by grants from the Medical Research Council of New Zealand and the National Children's Health Research Foundation of New Zealand (to Dr. J.S. Werry and Dr. M.G. Aman) and by a research project grant from the U.S. National Institute of Mental Health (Grant MH44122) to Dr. M.G. Aman.

References

Aman MG. (1978). Drugs, learning, and the psychotherapies. In JS Werry (ed.), *Pediatric psychopharmacology: The use of behavior modifying drugs in children* (pp. 79–108). New York: Brunner/Mazel.

Aman MG. Cognitive, social, and other correlates of specific reading retardation. *Journal of Abnormal Child Psychology*, 1979, 7:153–168.

Aman MG, Kern RA, McGhee D & Arnold LE. (1991a). *The effects of methylphenidate and fenfluramine on the behavior and cognitive performance of mentally retarded hyperactive children.* In preparation, Ohio State University, Columbus.

Aman MG, Marks RE, Turbott SH, Wilsher CP & Merry SN. Methylphenidate and thioridazine in intellectually subaverage children: Effects on cognitive-motor performance. *Journal of the American Academy of Child and Adolescent Psychiatry*, 1991b, 30:816–824.

Aman MG & Mayhew JM. Consistency of cognitive and motor performance measures over two years in reading retarded children. *Perceptual and Motor Skills*, 1980, 50:1059–1065.

Aman MG, Mitchell EA & Turbott SH. The effects of essential fatty acid supplementation by Efamol in hyperactive children. *Journal of Abnormal Child Psychology*, 1987a, 15:75–89.

Aman MG & Sprague RL. The state-dependent effects of methylphenidate and dextroamphetamine. *Journal of Nervous and Mental Diseases*, 1974, 158:268–279.

Aman MG & Turbott SH. Prediction of clinical response in children taking methylphenidate. *Journal of Autism and Developmental Disorders*, 1991, 21:211–227.

Aman MG, Vamos M & Werry JS. Effects of methlyphenidate in normal adults with reference to drug action in hyperactivity. *Australian and New Zealand Journal of Psychiatry*, 1984, 18:86–88.

Aman MG & Werry JS. Methylphenidate and diazepam in severe reading retardation. *Journal of the American Academy of Child Psychiatry*, 1982, 21:31–37.

Aman MG, Werry JS, Paxton JW & Turbott SH. Effects of sodium valproate on psychomotor performance in children as a function of dose, fluctuations in concentration, and diagnosis. *Epilepsia*, 1987b, 28:115–124.

Aman MG, Werry JS, Paxton JW & Turbott SH. (1991c). *Effects of phenytoin on psychomotor performance in children as a function of drug concentration, seizure type, and time of medication.* In preparation, The Ohio State University, Columbus.

Aman MG, Werry JS, Paxton JW, Turbott SH & Stewart AW. Effects of carbamazepine on psychomotor performance in children as a function of drug concentration, seizure type, and time of medication. *Epilepsia*, 1990, 31:51-60.

Birch HG & Belmont L. Auditory-visual integration in normal and retarded readers. *American Journal of Orthopsychiatry*, 1964, 34:852-861.

Blank M & Bridger WH. Deficiencies in verbal labeling in retarded readers. *American Journal of Orthopsychiatry*, 1966, 36:840-847.

Cull CA & Trimble MR. (1987). Automated testing and psychopharmacology. In: I Hineman & PD Storier (eds.), *Human psychopharmacology* (pp. 113-153). Chichester: John Wiley & Sons.

Cumming WW & Berryman R. (1965). The complex discriminated operant: Studies of matching-to-sample and related problems. In: DI Mostofsky (ed.), *Stimulus generalization* (pp. 284-330). Stanford: Stanford University Press.

Kagan J. (1965a). Impulsive and reflective children: Significance of conceptual tempo. In: JD Krumboltz (ed.), *Learning and the educational process* (pp. 133-161). Chicago: Rand McNally and Co.

Kagan J. Reflection-impulsivity and reading ability in primary grade children. *Child Development*, 1965b, 36:609-628.

Kløve H. Clinical neuropsychology. In: FM Forster (ed.), *The medical clinics of North America*, 1963, 47:1647-1658. New York: Saunders.

Scott KG. (1971). Recognition memory: A research strategy and summary of initial findings. In: NR Ellis (ed.), *International review of research in mental retardation* (vol. 5) (pp. 83-111). New York: Academic Press.

Sprague RL & Sleator EK. Effects of psychopharmacologic agents on learning disorders. *Pediatric Clinics of North America*, 1973, 20:719-735.

Sprague RL & Sleator EK. What is the proper dose of stimulant drugs in children? *International Journal of Mental Health*, 1975, 4:75-118.

Sprague RL & Sleator EK. Methylphenidate in hyperkinetic children: Differences in dose effects on learning and social behavior. *Science*, 1977, 198:1274-1276.

Sprague RL & Toppe LK. Relationship between activity level and delay of reinforcement. *Journal of Experimental Psychology*, 1966, 3:390-397.

Sternberg S. High-speed scanning in human memory. *Science*, 1966, 153:652-654.

Sykes D, Douglas V, Weiss G & Minde K. Attention in hyperactive children and the effect of methyphenidate (Ritalin). *Journal of Child Psychology and Psychiatry*, 1971, 12:129-139.

Werry JS & Aman MG. Methylphenidate and haloperidol in children. Effects on attention, memory, and activity. *Archives of General Psychiatry*, 1975, 32:790-795.

Werry JS & Aman MG. (1984). Methylphenidate in hyperactive and enuretic children. In: B Shopsin & L Greenhill (eds.), *The psychobiology of childhood: Profile of current issues* (pp. 183-195). Jamaica, NY: Spectrum Publications.

Werry JS, Aman MG & Diamond E. Imipramine and methylphenidate in hyperactive children. *Journal of Child Psychology and Psychiatry*, 1980, 21:27-35.

Werry JS, Elkind GS & Reeves JC. Attention deficit, conduct, oppositional, and anxiety disorders in children: III. Laboratory differences. *Journal of Abnormal Child Psychology*, 1987, 15:409–428.

6

Assessment of Mental Functions in Patients with Epilepsy: Cognitive Models and Ecological Constraints

Nicole von Steinbüchel and Ernst Pöppel

Institut für medizinische Psychologie, Ludwig-Maximilians-Universität München

Introduction

In the assessment of patients' mental functions the often divergent interests of the theoretically oriented scientist and the practitioner should be brought closer together. From the practical point of view it is essential to learn about the functional state of a patient in order to decide about possible therapeutic or rehabilitational measures. In contrast, the theorist often tries to define functional disturbances within a theoretical framework irrespective of the ecological constraints imposed by the activities of daily life. Notwithstanding, the practical demands in functional assessment may benefit from a theoretical perspective.

We hope to demonstrate that in the rather arbitrary selection of tests that appears to be guided by the more obvious deficits which patients show, one important domain of mental activities has been neglected—temporal control. Despite the fact that mental or motor speed is usually considered an important indicator for functional assessment (e.g., Dodrill 1978, 1988; Dodrill & Temkin 1989; Meador et al. 1990; Thompson et al. 1981; Reynolds 1983; Thompson & Trimble 1983; Trimble 1987) response latency obtained after defined stimulus presentations appears to be the only variable of interest. There is, however, more to temporal processing than is indicated by response times or speed measurements (e.g., Pöppel 1978, 1985) and a systematic evaluation of these temporal aspects may enhance knowledge about the functional status of patients with epilepsy.

One reason for the neglect of the temporal domain in the assessment of functions may be that the selection of tests is not guided by theory but by practical considerations or ecological constraints. As patients with epilepsy may demonstrate altered behavior or may report subjective phenomena, indicating disturbances in consciousness in general or in specific functional domains in particular (e.g., Gloor 1986; Penfield 1949), the selection of tests has been guided mainly by such reported deficits. Further, tests have been chosen with respect to their potential ability to detect problems in the activities of daily living (Dodrill 1978; Thompson et al. 1981; Trimble 1987). Thus, measures of attention, concentration, memory, problem solving, and motor and mental speed have been favored (see Kinsbourne and Lezak [this volume]).

The question, however, remains whether by concentrating on such "high level" cognitive functions the entire repertoire of functional competence is adequately represented. Obviously disturbances may occur on several levels of complexity including also "lower levels." A theoretical model might be useful to guide functional assessment. Therefore we present a theoretical attempt at cognitive modeling.

The Algorithmic Representation of Functions

If the monistic epistemological position is accepted that subjective phenomena can be described as brain states (Bunge 1980; Pöppel 1985 [1988]), neuropsychological observations, which indicate that specific lesions of the brain result in defined functional losses, can be used in this context. As it can be demonstrated that the destruction of circumscribed areas of the brain or specific neuronal algorithms leads to a loss of specific functions, it follows that under normal conditions these brain areas or algorithms are indispensable for these functions. Such a "modular" representation of functions has been amply verified (e.g., Damasio & Geschwind 1985). With respect to a potential classification of psychological functions one can draw the following conclusion: The entire repertoire of subjective phenomena is provided by distinct neuronal algorithms and each function is defined by its own neuronal algorithm. Thus a classification of psychological functions in such a biological approach is based on distinct brain mechanisms representing separate functions.

Beginning with Broca (1865) it has been demonstrated that specific functions are represented locally in the brain (Kertesz 1983). This principle of localization of function refers to four functional domains, namely (1) stimulus representation (perception), (2) stimulus processing (association, learning, and memory), (3) stimulus evaluation and assessment (emotion), and (4) stimulus response (action and reaction) (Gloor 1986; Pöppel 1989).

A few examples shall be given in order to indicate the principle of segregation of function, which for the class of stimulus representation, has been studied in most detail for the visual system (Zeki 1978). It can be demonstrated that specific visual functions are dependent on the integrity of circumscribed regions of the brain; if such regions are no longer in operation selective functions, such as seeing colors, recognizing faces, or perceiving movements are no longer available.

There are equivalent examples for the other sensory modalities and classes of psychological phenomena (Milner & Teuber 1968). It has been demonstrated that the mnemonic systems are organized in a modular fashion. Memory storage for instance is neuronally independent of recall, and procedural memory appears to be organized independent of referential memory.

For the class of stimulus evaluation also, segregation of function (i.e., the principle of modularity) seems to apply, as has for instance been demonstrated by brain stimulation experiments and by neuroethological observations. Different emotions are made available by distinct neuronal programs (Ploog 1980).

Finally, modularity can be assumed for the functions of action. One prominent example of this class of phenomena is speech. It can be demonstrated that different linguistic competences are based on the integrity of specific regions of the brain or generally speaking on particular neuronal algorithms.

The four functional domains referred to above are believed to comprise the content of the experiential repertoire. However, in order to obtain a subjective representation of mental phenomena, specific logistical requirements have to be met. For instance, without activation mental functions are not available; that is, they cannot reach the level of consciousness (Saper & Plum 1985). The circadian variation of activation as observed in the sleep–wakefulness cycle is one expression of the importance of activation but there may also be long-term modulations of activation like those due to the menstrual cycle or annual rhythms. The different attention mechanisms, such as selective or distributed attention, also belong to this class of logistical functions.

System States as Basis for Spatial and Temporal Binding

Given modularity: How are functions, which are represented by different neuronal algorithms, linked together? Further: How are elementary events in a successive order bound together to provide continuity of experience and the ordered sequence of mental events? It is suggested that specific types of system states provide the formal basis for binding operations (Pöppel et al. 1990a,b).

As described elsewhere (Pöppel 1985 [1988]), there is evidence for system states of approximately 30 to 40 msec duration. Experimental results suggest that stimuli that reach the sensory surface initiate excitability cycles or neuronal oscillations with a period that corresponds to the duration of these hypothetical system states (Pöppel 1968, 1970). A system state is characterized by the fact that temporal relationships between physical events within such a state cannot be defined; this implies that a system state of the brain corresponds to a zone of "atemporality" within which all available information is treated as cotemporaneous. We suggest that system states of 30 to 40 msec can be used as a logistical basis for binding operations. As the exact temporal central availability within such a time window does not seem to play a role, information from different regions of the brain and from different sense organs can be collected within such a time window. Thus the spatial segregation of functional representation can be overcome if system states are set up.

It is useful to distinguish between different levels of binding in order to indicate several different spatial and temporal binding operations. For the visual system, the lowest level of binding is presumably given by linking neuronal activities that represent identical features in different regions of the visual field (Gray et al. 1989). Such a binding may be presemantic and it may serve as a necessary prerequisite for the establishment of contours or surfaces throughout the visual field.

On the second level of binding the semantic domain is reached. If different qualities are to be linked together, such as contours, colors, and surfaces that define the perceived object the perceptual system has to select in a top-down manner which qualities have to be bound together. Thus a scheme of the perceived object has to be available. New evidence using PET-Scans (Corbetta et al. 1990) indicates that selective attention mechanisms working in a top-down model select spatially distributed brain regions, which as a pattern, are different for different attentional foci.

On the third level of binding information from different sensory channels has to be linked together. Objects in the world can be defined by information from different sense modalities, that is, by visual, auditory, olfactory, and tactile input. For intersensory integration a different neuronal mechanism has to be assumed than for intrasensory binding. It is an open question whether for intersensory binding a specific order has to be met in which information from different channels can be integrated within a contemporaneous operation.

Although these three levels of binding reviewed above may require different neuronal algorithms, theoretically it appears to be possible that system states with the duration of approximately 30 to 40 msec may be used as a logistical basis within which the binding operations can be implemented (Pöppel et al. 1990a,b). It has been pointed out in the special case of speech perception (von Steinbüchel & Pöppel 1991) that the combinatorical constraints are such that spatially distributed activities within system states can be easily represented in connectionistic networks.

Support for the notion of system states of the order of approximately 30 to 40 msec derives from various experimental paradigms. Multimodal histograms of choice reaction time suggest a discrete time sampling of the indicated duration (Harter & White 1968; Pöppel 1968, 1970). Studies on temporal-order threshold for different sense modalities suggest time quanta of approximately

30 msec duration (Hirsh & Sherrick 1961). Temporal order judgments appear to be very sensitive to cerebral disturbances (Swisher & Hirsh 1972; von Steinbüchel 1987). Further, oscillatory responses in auditory evoked potentials indicate an equivalent process of temporal segmentation (Galambos et al. 1981; Basar et al. 1987; Madler & Pöppel 1987; Madler et al. 1991). Interestingly, a temporal segmentation process of this duration is also suggested by single-cell recordings in the somatosensory system (Gardner & Costanzo 1980).

On a hierarchically higher level a further binding operation has to be suspected. It is characteristic for human perception, cognition or action that successive events—hearing a musical motif, processing visual motion, or uttering a phrase—are linked together. Experimentally, one can observe temporal integration processes that bind successive events together up to intervals of a few seconds (Pöppel 1978, 1985 [1988]). On an even higher level of binding, contents of consciousness are linked together. The integration intervals of a few seconds may serve as a formal basis to represent information, but as an operational prerequisite they do not determine "what" is represented and "how" the represented information is temporally linked together. The continuity of experience can be thought of being the result of a semantic connection of what is represented within successive integration intervals (Pöppel 1989).

Consequences for Functional Assessment

Before deriving some practical consequences for functional assessment we shall summarize the major points of the classificatory system outlined above. Two functional classes can be distinguished, the "what" functions that provide the content of experience, and the "how" functions that are responsible for the availability of functions. Within the class of "what" functions four domains have been distinguished—namely perception, processing, emotional evaluation, and action. The "what" functions are postulated to be based on particular neuronal modules or algorithms that may be localized, but not necessarily so. Two domains of "how" functions have to be distinguished—namely activation (including the different attention mechanisms) and temporal organization. Within the domain of temporal organization different binding operations have been identified that are located in different time domains: (1) a high frequency mechanism, responsible for rather short system states; (2) a low frequency mechanism that accounts for temporal integration up to a few seconds; and (3) a semantic linkage mechanism that accounts for the subjective continuity of mental activity. Several conclusions for a functional assessment can be drawn from this classificatory system of mental functions.

One conclusion is that functional assessment should cover all the domains in a representative fashion. Thus, specific tests have to be selected for perceptual, processing, evaluative or response functions and in addition for the logistical functions such as activation or attention and the different binding operations.

Yet in practice the entire repertoire of elementary "what" and "how" functions cannot be tested appropriately because this would take too long. One simply has to consider the tests necessary to assess all possible perceptual functions: Tests would have to be chosen for the different sensory modalities and also for the different qualities within these modalities. A comprehensive survey of perceptual functions alone would be too time consuming.

It follows from the practical constraints that functional competence of patients with epilepsy can only be sampled. For such a sampling it would be necessary that the selected tests are representative. Despite the impressive work on neuropsychological assessment in patients with epilepsy presented by many researchers (e.g., Reynolds 1983; Dodrill 1978, 1988; Thompson et al. 1981; Trimble 1987), it appears that criteria for the selection of representative tests still have to be found. At present, tests used for a neuropsychological evaluation of functions are chosen on the basis of clinical experience and statistical arguments. This results in an assessment of some functional domains, such as "measures of attention, representation of new information, speed and accuracy of perceptual registration, decision-making, and manual speed" (Trimble 1987), which are measured partly because they may appear "interesting and meaningful for patients and not time-consuming to complete" (Trimble 1987). Although these practical constraints are important we recommend that in future research the development of criteria for the selection of representative tests should be emphasized. The theoretical demand to use a test sample possibly representing all mental functions is opposed by the pragmatic necessity to test only those functions that show ecological validity. But how do elementary functions that characterize the "what" and the "how" of mental life map onto ecological relevant functions, such as reading, typing, or driving a car? To answer this must be an aim of future research.

At present, selection criteria for particular tests mainly depend on the specific assessment demands. Out of the entire repertoire of potential disturbances (e.g., Porter 1989) or a partial set of such disturbances as diagnosed in complex partial seizures (e.g., Bear 1979), different samples of tests for functional assessments are drawn stressing different domains of functional competence. This sampling of tests, however, is oriented toward practical constraints. If an assessment is performed by computerized tests, the selection of tests is biased toward those in which exact time control is dominant, like measuring response times. For evaluation of drug effects, for example (i.e., comparing different drugs or different dosages of one drug), the guiding principle for the test selection has to be to choose those that promise to be sensitive even for subtle effects. As such effects may only be detectable in a long-term comparison the possibility to apply tests several times or to monitor performance continuously must be available; that is, the practice effect for such tests has to be minimal. From a practical point of view, it is also important to choose those tests that do not take too long to be completed. To capture interest and to sustain necessary motivation of the patient entails a choice of those tests that are not too monotonous; compliance may otherwise become a problem.

The guiding principle of the selection of representative tests seems different given a theoretical orientation. At first, the decision has to be made as to which functional domains have to be monitored and in what way. The classificatory system presented above may be used as a potential guideline to define the sample of tests. As this taxonomy is of a general nature it applies also to diseases other than epilepsy. For example, it proved to be useful for the functional assessment of brain injury (Pöppel & von Steinbüchel 1991). For an assessment of cognitive functions it also has to be taken into account that "high-level functions" may be disturbed if "low-level functions" are affected (Milner & Teuber 1968); thus the assessment of elementary functions seems useful. At present, there is a strong bias in epileptology to assess mainly "high-level" cognitive functions: interestingly, in the motor domain "low-level" functions like tapping are favored. In the perceptual domain it may be useful to assess the different sensory modalities with the help of psychophysical measurements. In particular, the assessment of visual and auditory as well as tactile and especially olfactory perceptual thresholds seems useful, as perceptual alterations are characteristic events for certain seizures and may have a strong impact on the mood state.

Whereas the domains of learning and memory, and of volitional action and motor control are usually well represented in neuropsychological test batteries, the emotional evaluation of subjective phenomena appears to be under-represented. Using questionnaires for self-report of emotional alterations as well as behavioral measures by others may serve as a more complete assessment.

Within the domain of executive functions most test batteries emphasize the assessment of vigilance, attention, and mental speed. As mentioned above, measurements of temporal organization as expressed in the different binding operations are, however, neglected. As these temporal mechanisms are basic for cognitive processes they should be included in functional assessments. We would like to indicate three different classes of experimental procedures that allow a better appreciation of these basic central timing operations.

Examples for Functional Assessment

Measuring temporal-order threshold may allow an estimation of the time zone within which information is treated as simultaneous (Hirsh & Sherrick 1961; Swisher & Hirsh 1972; von Steinbüchel 1987). Dissociations of order thresholds in different sense modalities can be meaningful with respect to alterations of central information processing. The high correlation between temporal-order threshold and other experimental variables, such as the period of the mid-latency response of the auditory evoked potential (e.g., Galambos et al. 1981) or the intermodal distance in histograms of choice reaction times (e.g., Pöppel 1970) suggests that a single underlying mechanism is tapped which is essential for cerebral information processing. Should temporal-order threshold prove to be different for the different sensory channels, problems of intersensory integration may result. Alterations of "high-level" processing functions as measured for example by mental speed factors, may be related to disturbances on this lower level of temporal processing.

Simple and choice reaction time measurements are used in most test batteries of neuropsychological functional assessments. Despite this, an improved use of the variable appears still to be possible. As already mentioned, choice reaction time histograms often show a bimodal characteristic (e.g., Harter & White 1978; Pöppel 1968, 1970; Pöppel et al. 1990c). The bimodalities or multi-modalities are an expression of a discrete central time sampling, each mode within the response histogram indicating the discrete time toward which a response is attracted. These response characteristics have been explained on the basis of central neuronal oscillations that are triggered by sensory stimuli (Pöppel 1970; Tononi et al. 1991). Interhemispheric intra- and intersensory choice reaction time can be considered as a paradigm that provides answers to the question of the estimation of mental and motor speed. If the GO reaction is measured, central decision times and movement times can be estimated independently (Steinbach et al. 1991). In a Go reaction the release of a response key after stimulus presentation is defined as *reaction time*, whereas the time between release and reaching a decision key is defined as *movement time*. This could be useful if drug effects on mental and motor speed have to be evaluated. As the task of intrahemispheric choice reaction time is rather demanding, learning curves can be obtained separately for information processing in the two hemispheres. In addition, the variance of responses is an excellent indicator of the patient's ability to maintain concentration throughout the test session.

Whereas measurements of temporal-order threshold and choice reaction time give some insight into high frequency mechanisms of temporal information processing, additional tests may allow the proper assessment of low frequency mechanism of temporal integration. It has been demonstrated that successive sensory information is bound together up to intervals of a few seconds (Pöppel 1978, 1985 [1988]; Schleidt et al. 1987). Temporal integration in this time domain appears to be an automatic process related to basic operations of the mental machinery. This model suggests that mental operations are segmented in time each segment lasting only a few seconds. Thus, the subjective continuity apparent on the experiential level appears to be due to semantic linkage of "what" is represented within such time segments; the representational process itself, however, is discrete in nature. As this seems to be a rather basic process in cognition it appears to be useful to obtain objective measurements in epileptic patients.

It has already been demonstrated that after local brain injuries (Pöppel et al. 1978), temporal integration may be disturbed. Using a simple tapping test may quickly give information about a patient's capacity to integrate information. Auditory stimuli are presented in a regular fashion and the patient's task is to synchronize his or her taps with the stimulus sequence. If the inter-stimulus-interval (ISI) is short, the subject anticipates the stimulus occurrence by some tens of milliseconds; this anticipation is often characterized by a multimodal distribution of movement initiations with a temporal interval distance of approximately 30 msec (Radil et al. 1990). This phenomenon of stimulus anticipation is observed for ISIs up to 2 to 3 s. If the ISI is greater, subjects can no longer anticipate. In this case each stimulus of the sequence elicits a reaction; that is, actually simple reaction time is measured. This test allows an easy estimation of temporal binding operations, and it remains to be investigated whether in patients with epilepsy this basic logistical operation is altered or whether it is affected by certain drug treatments.

The tests referred to above are suggested as complementary to the existing neuropsychological test batteries. They are derived from a neuropsychological classification of functions. It can be expected that functional assessment of patients with epilepsy would benefit from such a theoretical orientation.

Acknowledgments

Research of the authors referred to here was supported by the Deutsche Forschungsgemeinschaft and the Bundesminister für Forschung und Technologie.

References

Basar E, Rosen B, Basar-Eroglu C & Greitschus F. The associations between 40 Hz-EEG and the middle latency response of the auditory evoked potential. *International Journal of Neuroscience*, 1987, 33:103–117.

Bear DM. (1979). The temporal lobes: An approach to the study of organic behavioral change. In: MS Gazzaniga (ed.), *Handbook of behavioral neurobiology* (vol. 2): *Neuropsychology* (pp. 75–95). New York: Plenum Press.

Broca P. Sur le Siège de la Faculté du Langage Articulé. *Bull. Soc. Anthropol.*, 1865, 337–393.

Bunge M. (1980). *The mind-body problem: A psychobiological approach*. Oxford: Pergamon Press.

Corbetta M, Miezin FM, Dobmeyer S, Shulman GL & Peterson SE. Attentional modulation of neural processing of shape, color, and velocity in humans. *Science*, 1990, 248:1556–1559.

Damasio AR & Geschwind N. (1985). Anatomical localization in clinical neuropsychology. In: JAM Frederiks (ed.), *Handbook of clinical neurology* (vol. 1): *Clinical neuropsychology* (pp. 7–22). Amsterdam: Elsevier.

Dodrill CB. A neuropsychological battery for epilepsy. *Epilepsia*, 1978, 19:611-623.
Dodrill CB. (1988). Neuropsychology. In: J Laidlaw, A Richens & J Oxley (eds.), *A textbook of epilepsy* (pp. 406-420). New York: Churchill Livingstone.
Dodrill CB & Temkin NR. Motor speed is a contaminating factor in evaluating the "cognitive" effects of phenytoin. *Epilepsia*, 1989, 30:453-457.
Galambos R, Makeig S & Talmachoff PJ. A 40-Hz auditory potential recorded from the human scalp. *Proc. Nat. Acad. Science U.S.A.*, 1981, 78:2643-2647.
Gardner EP & Costanzo RM. Temporal integration of multipoint stimuli in primary somatosensory cortical receptive fields of alert monkeys. *Journal of Neurophysiology*, 1980, 43:444-468.
Gloor P. Consciousness as a neurological concept in epileptology: A critical review. *Epilepsia*, 1986, 27 (suppl. 2):S14-S26.
Gray CM, König P, Engel AK & Singer W. Oscillatory responses in cat visual cortex exhibit inter-columnar synchronization which reflects global stimulus properties. *Nature*, 1989, 338:334-337.
Harter R & White CT. Periodicity within reaction time distributions and electromyograms. *Quarterly Journal Experimental Psychology*, 1968, 20:157-166.
Hirsh IJ & Sherrick CE Jr. Perceived order in different sense modalities. *Journal of Exper. Psychol.*, 1961, 62:423-432.
Kertesz, A. (1983). Issues in localization. In: A Kertesz (ed.), *Localisation in neuropsychology* (pp. 287-331). Amsterdam: Elsevier.
Madler A & Pöppel E. Auditory evoked potentials indicate the loss of neuronal oscillations during general anaesthesia. *Naturwissenschaften*, 1987, 74:42-43.
Madler C, Keller I, Schwender D & Pöppel E. Sensory information processing during general anaesthesia: Effects of isoflurane on auditory evoked neuronal oscillations. *Brit. Journ. Anaesthesia*, 1991, 66: 81-87.
Meador KJ, Loring DW, Huh K, Gallagher BB & King DW. Comparative cognitive effects of anticonvulsants. *Neurology*, 1990, 40:391-394.
Milner B & Teuber H-L. (1968). Alteration of perception and memory in man: Reflections on method. In: L Weiskrantz (ed.), *Analysis of behavioral change* (pp. 268-375). New York: Harper and Row.
Penfield W. Epileptic manifestations of cortical and supracortical discharge. *Electroencephalography and Clinical Neurophysiology*, 1949, 1:3-10.
Ploog D. Emotionen als Produkte des limbischen Systems. *Medizinische Psychologie*, 1980, 6:7-19.
Pöppel E. Oszillatorische Komponenten in Reaktionszeiten. *Naturwissenschaften*, 1968, 55:449-450.
Pöppel E. Excitability cycles in central intermittency. *Psychologische Forschung*, 1970, 34:1-9.
Pöppel E. (1978). Time perception. In: R Held, H Leibowitz & H-L Teuber (eds.), *Handbook of sensory physiology* (vol. VIII): *Perception* (pp. 713-729). Berlin: Springer-Verlag.
Pöppel E. (1985 [1988]). *Grenzen des βewußtseins. Über Wirklichkeit und Welterfahrung*. Stuttgart: Deutsche Verlagsanstalt. English version: *Mindworks, time and conscious experience*. New York: Harcourt Brace Jovanovich.
Pöppel E. (1989). Taxonomy of the subjective: An evolutionary perspective. In: JW Brown (ed.), *Neuropsychology of visual perception*. Hillsdale, NJ: Erlbaum.

Pöppel E, Brinkmann R, von Cramon D & Singer W. Association and dissociation of visual functions in a case of bilateral occipital lobe infarction. *Archiv für Psychiatri Nervenkrankheiten*, 1978, 225:1–21.

Pöppel E, Ruhnau E, Schill K & von Steinbüchel N. (1990a). A hypothesis concerning timing in the brain. In: H Haken & M Stadler (eds.), *Synergetics in cognition* (pp. 144–149). Berlin: Springer.

Pöppel E, Schill K & von Steinbüchel N. Sensory integration within temporally neutral system states: A hypothesis. *Naturwissenschaften*, 1990b, 77:89–91.

Pöppel E, Schill K & von Steinbüchel N. Multistable states in intrahemispheric learning of a sensorimotor task. *Neuroreport*, 1990c, 1:69–72.

Pöppel E & von Steinbüchel N. (1991, in press). Neuropsychological rehabilitation from a theoretical point of view. In: N von Steinbüchel, D von Cramon & E Pöppel (eds.), *Neuropsychological rehabilitation*. Heidelberg: Springer-Verlag.

Porter RJ. (1989). *Epilepsy: 100 elementary principles*. London: W.B. Saunders.

Radil T, Mates J, Ilmberger J & Pöppel E. Stimulus anticipation in following rhythmic acoustical patterns by tapping. *Experientia*, 1990, 46:762–763.

Reynolds EH. Mental effects of antiepileptic medication: A review. *Epilepsia*, 1983, (suppl. 2) 24:S85–S95.

Saper CP & Plum F. (1985). Disorders of consciousness. In: JAM Frederiks (ed.), *Handbook of clinical neurology*, Vol. 1 (45): *Clinical neuropsychology* (pp. 107–128). Amsterdam: Elsevier.

Schleidt M, Eibl-Eibelsfeldt I & Pöppel E. A universal constant in temporal segmentation of human short-term behaviour. *Naturwissenschaften*, 1987, 74:289–290.

Steinbach Th, von Dreden G & Pöppel E. Long-term training in a choice reaction time task reveals different learning characteristics for the visual and auditory system. *Naturwissenschaften*, 1991, 78:185–187.

Swisher L & Hirsh I. Brain damage and ordering of two temporally successive stimuli. *Neuropsychologia*, 1972, 10:135–152.

Thompson P, Huppert FA & Trimble M. Phenytoin and cognitive function: Effects on normal volunteers and implications for epilepsy. *Brit. Journ. of Clinic. Psychol.*, 1981, 20:155–162.

Thompson P & Trimble MR. The effect of anticonvulsant drugs on cognitive function: Relation to serum levels. *Journ. Neurol. Neurosurg. Psychiatry*, 1983, 46:277–283.

Tononi G, Sporns D, Edelman GM. (1991, in press). The problem of neural integration: Induced rhythms and short-term correlations. In: E Basar & T Bullock (eds.), *Induced rhythms*.

Trimble MR. Anticonvulsant drugs and cognitive function: A review of the literature. *Epilepsia* (suppl. 3), 1987, 28:S37–S45.

von Steinbüchel N. (1987). Therapie der zeitlichen Verarbeitung akustischer Reize bei aphasischen Patienten. Unpublished dissertation, Medical Faculty Munich.

von Steinbüchel N & Pöppel E. (1991). Temporal order threshold and language perception. In: VP Bhatkar & KM Rege (eds.), *Frontiers in knowledge-based computing* (pp. 81–90). New Delhi: Narosa Publ. House.

Zeki S. Functional specialisation in the visual cortex of the rhesus monkey. *Nature*, 1978, 274:423–428.

—— **7** ——

Computer-Assisted Neuropsychological Assessment in Patients with Epilepsy

A–L. Rugland, O. Henriksen, and H. Bjørnœs

The National Center for Epilepsy
Sandvika, Norway

Introduction

The use of computers in psychological testing and assessment has increased tremendously since the introduction of the user-friendly microcomputers and software. The market is swiftly expanding for automated test-scoring services, computerized test interpretation, computer-administered tests, and software to perform these functions. To these technological innovations, the users and developers must apply the same professional and technical standards that govern the traditional means of performing these functions. The traditional neuropsychological tests are still in common use and cannot be fully replaced by computerized tests.

The application of computer technology is no better than the decision rules or algorithms upon which they are based. However, some aspects of testing can be carried out advantageously by a computer. The condition of administration of some tests can be better standardized and more accurately timed and controlled when the test is administered by a computer. Test scoring can be achieved more efficiently and accurately by a computer than it can manually. Test-score interpretation based on complex decision rules can be generated quickly and accurately by a computer. Further, the level of difficulty and duration of a test session can more readily be adjusted to an individual patient and learning effects more easily avoided by programs that present stimuli in a randomized order.

The Use of Computer-Assisted
Neuropsychological Tests in Patients with Epilepsy

Computerization of traditional neuropsychological tests may be of great value in assessing cognitive functioning in patients with epilepsy (Alpherts & Aldenkamp 1990). Some of these patients, however, have special problems that require tests especially constructed for this group. Three such problem areas will be described here: (1) the effect of subclinical epileptogenic EEG discharges on cognition; (2) adjustment of antiepileptic drug doses in patients who are impaired on test performance during epileptogenic EEG discharges; and (3) evaluation of the effect of stimulant medication in children with attention-deficit disorder.

At the National Center for Epilepsy (in Norway) we have been concerned by the fact that many patients with epilepsy continue to have serious problems with attention, concentration, and learning even after clinical seizures have been eliminated and only subclinical EEG discharges persist. We would like to know whether or not such discharges might be one of the causes for learning and behavioral problems. We have therefore developed a computerized neuropsychological test battery combined with simultaneous EEG registration making possible direct visual inspection of test performance in relation to the EEG.

Because most of the traditional neuropsychological tests are unsuitable for the extended and repeated testing necessary for evaluating the impact of subclinical EEG discharges on cognitive function, we started the development and assembling of the Rugland neuropsychological test battery in 1984 (Rugland et al. 1987). This battery fulfills the following criteria:

1. The tests are automatically administered.
2. Video monitoring is always performed during baseline and testing to detect subtle clinical manifestations to EEG discharges. Such instances are eliminated from the statistical analysis because they are not subclinical according to our operational definition.
3. The system has an exact event marking on the EEG record to allow direct comparison of performance in periods with and without discharges.
4. The tests allow for manipulation of several parameters, such as stimulus exposure time, and level of difficulty. Although the test parameters are kept constant in as many patients as possible, we have to adjust some of them according to the patient's mental capacity.
5. The test items are randomized by the computer to minimize practice effects, thus making multiple retesting more appropriate.

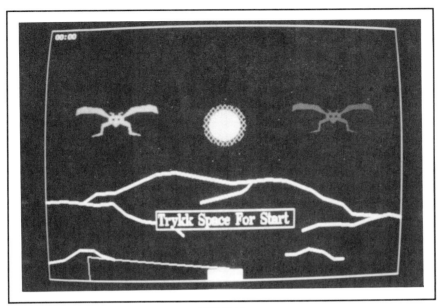

FIGURE 1

The introduction picture of the choice reaction time test where the patients are told that red space monsters are to be shot down while the sun and space monsters in colors other than red are not to be responded to.

6. Some of the tests are constructed to give material-specific information on lateralization and location of cognitive function (i.e., verbal versus figurative tasks).

7. The tests are relevant to some cognitive functions that seem impaired in patients with epilepsy, such as concentration and memory.

8. The tests are applicable to patients with mental ages ranging from 5 years to adult.

9. Many of our patients are children who have to be tested for an extended time; therefore, efforts have been made to make the graphic designs appealing to children. For example, in the simple reaction time test there is a space monster to be shot down.

The Test Battery

The Rugland neuropsychological test battery was developed over a period of 4 years. For the past 3 years the battery has been used routinely for patients with subclinical EEG discharges. Several tests were developed but which were not incorporated in the final battery; only the most satisfactory have been included. The battery consists of the following tests:

1. The *Romny* tests are tests that consist of a simple reaction time test (Romny 1) and two choice reaction time tests—Romny 2 or 3—depending on the patient's age or mental capacity. During the simple reaction time test a response to an unambiguous stimulus, a red space monster is required. The stimulus is delivered at irregular intervals ranging from 0.5 to 1.5 s over a period of 5 m. During the choice reaction time test the patient alternates between responding to a red space monster and not responding during the presentation of a sun or space monsters in colors other than red. The stimuli are delivered according to the same procedure as the simple reaction time test. The test lasts for 10 m. These tests are intended to measure mental and psychomotor speed as well as attention. This implies selective response to a given stimulus or stimuli; and vigilance, which refers to general reactivity of the organism to incoming stimuli.

2. The *Corsi* tests consist of a verbal and nonverbal topographic and spatial short-term memory test; and may also be defined as verbal and topographic memory span tests. The memory function is tested immediately after the presentation of the material. The Corsi tests have kindly been received from Dr. Binnie and his coworkers at the Instituut voor Epilepsiebestrijding, Heemstede in the Netherlands. The topographic task has some similarity to Corsi's block test (Milner 1971). More detailed description of these tests has been given by Aarts et al. (1984). Each test is run for 10 m.

3. The *Ranton* tests consist of a verbal and a figurative problem-solving test. The instruction is simple: Point to the word or figure that differs in some way from the others (oddity problems). The tests contain 6 levels of difficulty, which require an increasing ability to form abstract rules. When 5 correct responses are given, a higher level of complexity is automatically introduced whereas 3 incorrect responses lead to a lower level of complexity. The sessions start with the presentation of 3 items, ending with 5 in the verbal test and 6 in the figurative test at the most complex level.

The performances between and during discharges are compared by means of a 2 × 2 contingency table showing the incidence of correct and incorrect responding during the two conditions. Until now the test battery has been used in N-1 designs only, such that each patient is his or her own control. However, to obtain a basis for a wider generalization, the computerized tests have now been validated against traditional neuropsychological measures. Test–retest effects have been investigated (reliability) and norms are collected from normal controls. The results between different groups of patients with epilepsy will be established.

Cognitive Dysfunction and Subclinical Epileptogenic Activity

The fact that subclinical EEG discharges may disturb cognitive functioning in patients with epilepsy was recognized a long time ago. In 1939, Schwab demonstrated that when patients performed a simple reaction time task during EEG monitoring, spike-wave discharges might be accompanied by slowed reaction or indeed a complete failure to respond. Since that time, more than 40 additional studies have investigated this phenomenon (Aarts et al. 1984).

The results of these studies are quite consistent with only a few exceptions. Most investigators have found impaired performance during subclinical spike-wave discharges in about half the patients studied. The reports indicate that performance during mentally demanding tasks are influenced to a greater extent than simple, more automatic responses such as finger tapping, counting, recitation, and simple reaction time. Impaired performance seems related to specific EEG phenomena and is most easily observed during generalized symmetrical regular spike-wave discharges that last 3 s or more. However, Aarts et al. (1984) found that there was an interaction between the nature of the task and lateralization of discharges. As will be discussed below, even focal discharges of 1 s or less sometimes impairs performance (Rugland et al. 1987; Rugland 1990).

In one study (25 children, 24 adults) we found that during testing epileptogenic activity decreased in 45% and increased in 16% of the patients, compared with a relaxed baseline period (Rugland et al. 1987; Rugland 1990). Thus, in some patients increased concentration during testing reduces ongoing epileptogenic activity whereas in others the stress in a test situation increases the discharge rate. Significant impairment of performance during discharges was seen in 61% of the patients on either a simple reaction time test, a choice reaction time test, or both. In patients with generalized discharges, 67% showed impaired performance compared to only 33% of patients with focal or markedly asymmetrical discharges.

In 1983, 31 children with subclinical EEG discharges in their standard EEG were referred for neuropsychological testing combined with EEG registration. Of these, 26 children had serious academic problems; 3 had minor problems; and only 2 had no reported school problems. Although learning problems were not a particular criterion for this investigation, the clinicians often mentioned this in their referral. Twelve of the children had too few discharges to allow statistical analysis and 2 were excluded because of clinically visible absence seizures. Of the remaining 17 children, 15 were affected on one or more tests by the subclinical discharges in their EEGs.

Figure 2 shows an example of the EEG record during testing in a 10-year-old girl. As can be seen, she performed quite well in periods without discharges whereas her performance deteriorated during epileptogenic discharges. All 15 children (except one) had academic problems. Although many psychological factors may influence these children's learning ability, there is growing evidence that subclinical EEG discharges play an important role (Kasteleijen-Nolst Trenité et al. 1988; Seidenberg et al. 1988; Siebelink et al. 1988). There is no reason to believe that impairment of memory and concentration caused by subclinical EEG discharges in the laboratory is any different from similar disturbances in school.

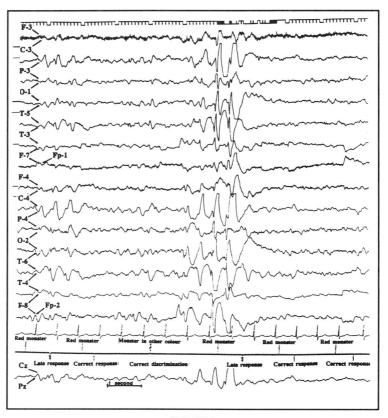

FIGURE 2

Epileptogenic EEG discharges during choice reaction time performance. The marker channel (16) indicates stimuli (marks upward) and responses (marks downward). During periods without discharges the patient is responding correctly whereas during discharges she is responding too late, that is, after the stimulus has disappeared.

The video recording from the test situation may also be used therapeutically. A child's self-image sometimes benefits by showing the child how well he or she performs when there are no discharges in the EEG. Children learn to recognize that they are not stupid and that their problems are related to the EEG discharges. One may also show them that the frequency of subclinical discharges may be drastically reduced when they concentrate, or that the discharge rate increases when they become tired. In this way they may be trained to be more aware of the signals from their body and learn to better cope with the problems related to subclinical EEG discharges. When the video recording of a child's performance during testing is shown to parents and teachers, they frequently express a new understanding of the child's otherwise strange behavior. Marked improvement in the interaction between parents and children has been obtained by this process. In school, an individually tailored program helps to improve the learning situation for these children.

Individual Effects of Subclinical EEG Discharges

Individuals differ exclusively in impairment on test performances during subclinical EEG discharges. To reveal impairment during EEG discharges it is important that different kinds of tests covering different cognitive functions are administered. This may be illustrated by the test results on 3 patients.

Patient 1 has very short epileptogenic discharges in the EEG that vary from 0.2 to 2.0 s duration. The frequency of discharges was moderate (mean 0.5 per minute) during the baseline period. The discharges were focal over the right hemisphere with a tendency to generalize. There was a fivefold increase in discharge frequency during the complex problem-solving tests (mean 2.6 per minute). This child's performance was significantly disturbed by the EEG discharges only during the verbal problem solving test.

Patient 2 had frequent EEG discharges (8.9 per minute) with a duration varying from 0.2 to 7.5 s during the baseline period. There was a moderate

Patient 1

TASKS:	RESULTS				x^2 - test (p-values)
	Number correct		Number wrong		
	With discharges	Without disch.	With discharges	Without disch.	
Baseline	-	-	-	-	-
Reaction time	*	*	*	*	*
Choice reaction time	*	*	*	*	*
Spatial memory	6	31	5	21	ns
Verbal memory	4	24	4	25	ns
Figurative problem solving	6	33	7	12	ns
Verbal problem solving	2	9	15	11	0.05

* Too few discharges to allow statistical analysis

FIGURE 3a

Test performance on a simple reaction time test, a choice reaction time test, a topographic and spatial short-term memory test, a verbal short-term memory test, a figurative problem-solving test, and a verbal problem-solving test during periods with and without epileptogenic EEG discharges. Patient 1's performance is impaired on the verbal problem-solving test only.

Patient 2

TASKS:	RESULTS				x^2 - test (p-values)
	Number correct		Number wrong		
	With discharges	Without disch.	With discharges	Without disch.	
Baseline	-	-	-	-	-
Reaction time	16	91	1	10	ns
Choice reaction time	40	152	11	20	0.05
Spatial memory	10	12	13	3	0.05
Verbal memory	10	7	12	0	0.01*
Figurative problem solving	17	26	9	4	ns
Verbal problem solving	15	27	13	1	0.01

*Fisher exact probability test

FIGURE 3b

Test performance on the same tests as described in Figure 3a during periods with and without epileptogenic EEG discharges. Patient 2's performance is impaired on the choice reaction time test, the topographic short-term memory test, the verbal short-term memory test, and the verbal problem-solving test. The most pronounced impairment is seen on the verbal tests.

Patient 3

TASKS:	RESULTS				x^2 - test (p-values)
	Number correct		Number wrong		
	With discharges	Without disch.	With discharges	Without disch.	
Baseline	-	-	-	-	-
Reaction time	14	66	20	11	0.01
Choice reaction time	10	112	16	66	0.01
Spatial memory	2	24	3	17	ns
Verbal memory	4	13	7	6	ns
Figurative problem solving	13	26	11	8	0.05
Verbal problem solving	7	27	4	10	ns

FIGURE 3c

Test performance on the same tests as described in Figure 3a during periods with and without epileptogenic EEG discharges. Patient 3's performance is impaired on the simple reaction time test, the choice reaction time test, and the figurative problem-solving test. The most pronounced impairment is seen on the reaction time tests.

decrease both in frequency and duration of the discharges during testing. EEG showed focal spike-wave activity in the right more than the left temporal lobe. There were also occasional bursts of polyspikes. The patient's performance was impaired by the EEG discharges on all the tests except during the simple reaction time test and during the figurative problem-solving test.

Patient 3 had very long-lasting discharges (varying from 4.5 to 73.5 s) during the baseline period. The discharge frequency was moderate averaging 0.9 per minute during baseline. The duration—but not the frequency—decreased dramatically during testing (varying from 1.5 to 21.0 s). The EEG showed bilaterally synchronous atypical spike-wave complexes, more or less generalized. In contrast to what one would expect, this patient was impaired on the simple reaction time test, the choice reaction time test, and on the figurative problem-solving test but not on other complex tasks. The impairment was most pronounced during the reaction time tests indicating a slowing of motor speed.

Patient 3 illustrates a phenomenon that is sometimes seen in an EEG-video-telemetry laboratory. Some patients seem quite unaffected by frequent and relatively long-lasting spike-wave discharges. Although they talk and read apparently undisturbed, the performance during neuropsychological testing of the same patients is impaired. The talking/reading situation may, however, not be structured enough to reveal more subtle changes in speed and accuracy during discharges.

Task complexity influences the extent of impairment that is detected during epileptic discharges. Tizard and Margerison (1963a,b) showed that the effect of spike-wave discharges is not all or none but rather the effect is proportional to the information-processing demands of the task: The greater the amount of information presented per stimulus, the greater the impairment. This aspect may explain apparently contradictory findings of other authors who, on the one hand, have found little or no psychological impairment during spike-wave discharges (Prechtl et al. 1961) or who, on the other, have showed considerable impairment (Davidoff & Johnson 1964). In the former case, the average rate of information presented per stimulus was low; in the latter, it was high.

This, however, cannot fully explain the difference in all test results because one patient may be impaired in only one of several tests with apparently the same amount of information per stimulus. Aarts et al. (1984) found an interaction between the nature of the task and lateralization of discharges. Patients were more likely to display impairment on the spatial task if the focal discharge was lateralized to the right hemisphere and on verbal task if left sided. Thus, depending on the location of discharges, impairment is expected on different types of tests.

Both localization of discharges and the complexity of the test may be of importance for the demonstration of impairment. However, as seen above, these explanations do not necessarily hold for each individual patient. It is not always possible to demonstrate a causality between localized epileptogenic activity and specific performance, partly because of the limitation of scalp EEG, often recording at a long distance from the epileptic focus, and because of the limitation of the tests that are used.

Computerized Testing and Optimizing Medication

The Rugland neuropsychological test battery has been developed primarily as a clinical device. Along with being used for diagnostic purposes, such as revealing impairment caused by subclinical epileptogenic discharges, it is also used to adjust and optimize antiepileptic medication in patients who have disturbed test performances by EEG discharges. For this reason it is important to ascertain that the patients benefit from the medication by reducing the subclinical discharges without unacceptable side effects. The patients are first tested at subtherapeutic serum levels, then in mid-range, and finally at a high serum level with computerized testing accompanied by EEG and video recording. The medication is stabilized on each dose level, and the patient tested at intervals of 1–3 months. In this way, the optimal dose for each individual with respect to seizures, EEG discharges, as well as cognitive functioning can be established. A similar procedure is applied during discontinuation of medication when a patient has been without subclinical EEG discharges for 2 years.

An illustration of the application of this procedure in an 8-year-old girl is seen in Figures 4a, b, c, and d. The EEG showed more or less generalized spike-wave activity with a right sided preponderance. In addition there were

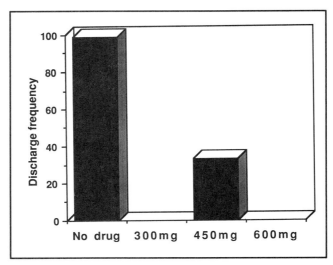

FIGURE 4a

The effect of different doses of valproate on epileptogenic EEG discharges in an 8-year-old girl during baseline and testing.

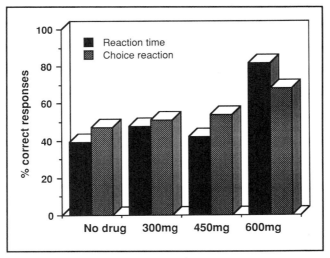

FIGURE 4b

The effect of different doses of valproate on a simple reaction time test and a choice reaction time test in an 8-year-old girl.

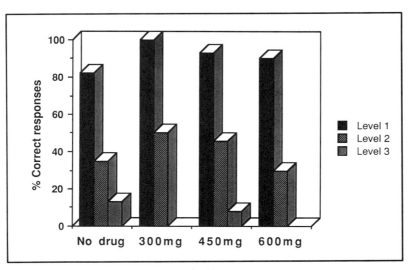

FIGURE 4c

The effect of different doses of valproate on a verbal short-term memory test with different levels of difficulty in an 8-year-old girl.

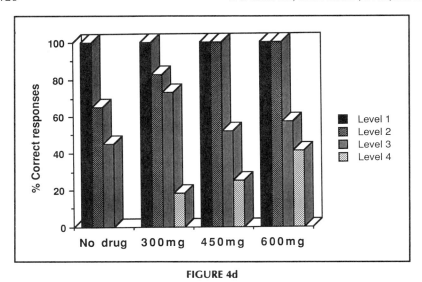

FIGURE 4d

The effect of different doses of valproate on a topographic short-term memory test with different levels of difficulty in an 8-year-old girl.

quite frequent theta-delta bursts. Here only the paroxysms with spike-wave activity are considered. The spike-wave bursts impaired her performance on all tests. She was tested on a low serum level—264 μmol/l, receiving 300 mg sodium valproate per day; in mid-range—479 μmol/l, receiving 450 mg sodium valproate per day; and on a relatively high serum level—572 μmol/l, receiving 600 mg sodium valproate per day. Figure 4a shows that there was an effect on the low dose of sodium valproate (300 mg) on the spike-wave activity that first disappeared only to reappear after some weeks. On the highest dose there was no spike-wave activity, but still frequent theta-delta bursts. Figure 4b shows the test results on the simple reaction time test and on the choice reaction time test. There is a marked improvement in test performance at the highest dose when epileptogenic EEG discharges are absent. However, this effect was not observed on 300 mg. Figures 4c and 4d show the results of the verbal memory task and of the topographic memory tasks on different doses respectively. In these tests the levels refer to difficulty: on level 1, one stimulus is presented; on level 2, two stimuli are presented, and so on. On 300 mg there is improvement especially on the nonverbal task. The most pronounced improvement of the performance is seen on the topographic task on 600 mg on level 4. On the verbal memory task, however, the performance seems to deteriorate somewhat, indicating an adverse effect of the medication. One may speculate whether these results were caused by the marked reduction of the pathology in the right hemisphere with increasing antiepileptic medication, while the left hemisphere initially less disturbed by the EEG discharges was impaired as side effects of the same drug administration. Both parents and the teacher of the child reported improved functioning both at school and at home on the highest dose but not on the lowest.

The effect of antiepileptic medication on subclinical EEG discharges as well as on performance varies from one person to another. Therefore the dose has to be adjusted to the individual. A decline in test results has been observed at a high serum level in some children. The reports from parents and teachers after an optimal dose is established are promising concerning school performance and/or behavior, but in a few cases a child may show clear improvement on test performance without any obvious changes in behavior at school or at home. It is important, however, to realize that a long history of inadequate behavior in some of these children cannot be changed overnight. When required, these children are supplied with a specially tailored learning program and psychological guidance at home.

Concentration Problems in Children with Epilepsy

Attention-deficit disorder with or without hyperactivity is occasionally seen in children with epilepsy. At our center some of these children are treated with

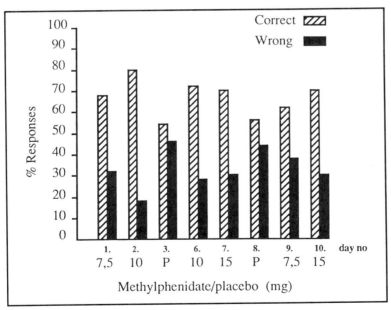

FIGURE 5

The test results from the blind testing with different doses of methylphenidate and placebo in a 6-year-old girl.

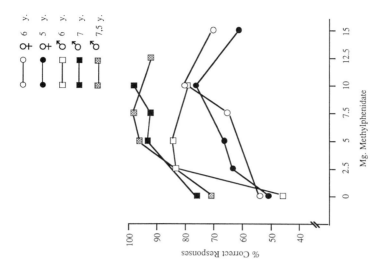

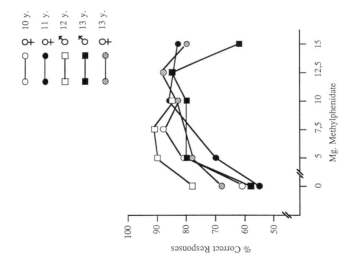

central stimulant medication (i.e., methylphenidate) when the diagnosis is established. To achieve a better (and more objective) evaluation of the effect of this medication the computerized choice reaction time test has been incorporated into a program of accurate observation and testing during a double-blind placebo versus drug administration.

In 1987 a pilot study was carried out on 20 children with concentration problems (Rugland & Bjørnœs 1987). Most of them were hyperactive as well. All the children had well-controlled seizures. The children were tested blindly twice 1 hour after intake of three different dosages of the drug or placebo. They were always tested at the same time of the day. The testing was combined with an EEG registration with video monitoring of the patient. After the test session the children were observed for 1 hour at school or in the ward, using a modification of Connors' (1969) scale.

Figure 5 shows the test results of the evaluation of a 6-year-old girl. As can be seen from this diagram, the dosages and placebo were given in a semi-randomized order to prevent sequence effects. The diagram shows that the child's performance improved during the administration of methylphenidate. More so than on the placebo days the child achieves about 25% less correct responses compared with the best day with medication. At 7.5 and 15.0 mg the test results are almost the same. Her best performance is achieved at 10 mg.

Ten children showed improvement in test performance and behavior on the drug. Figure 6a shows the individual test results on different dosages of the 5 youngest of these children (5 to 7 years) and Figure 6b the corresponding results for the 5 older ones (10 to 13 years). The diagrams show the individual dose-related change in performance. At the highest doses performance declines. Thus an inverted ∪-shape is seen in test performance with increasing dose of methylphenidate.

The characteristic test response pattern of these children when receiving placebo is errors of commission (i.e., depressing the response button when they should withhold the response to stimuli and also responding when no stimuli are presented). This indicates that the children have difficulty controlling impulses and withholding responses. When given methylphenidate this response pattern improves.

The test results were analyzed by means of a two-tailed student t-test. Because of few observations on some dosages, only the doses of 5–10 and 15 mg have been included in the analysis. The results show a statistically significant increase in % Correct Responses from baseline to 5 mg methylphenidate ($p < 0.01$) and from baseline to 10 mg ($p < 0.01$). At the 15 mg dose the conclusion is more uncertain because only 5 children have been tested. The statistical analysis shows no significant difference between baseline and 15 mg indicating a reduction in % Correct Responses compared with 5 and 10 mg dosages.

The results from this pilot study indicate that there may be different dose-response curves for different kinds of behavior because behavior improved on higher doses than the test performance. This confirms the results of Sprague and Sleator (1975).

Conclusion

The purpose of this presentation is to draw the attention to three areas on which computerized tests have contributed to the neuropsychological assessment in patients with epilepsy at our center. This approach is especially useful to evaluate the effect of subclinical EEG discharges on cognition. Cognitive side effects may be avoided by repeated testing on different doses of antiepileptic medication. The choice reaction time test is incorporated into an extensive program where children with serious concentration problems are tested blindly on a central stimulant drug. No doubt computerized test methods will become even more sophisticated in the future and the areas for their use will expand.

References

Aarts JHP, Binnie CD, Smit AN & Wilkins AJ. Selective cognitive impairment during focal and generalized epileptiform EEG activity. *Brain*, 1984, 107:293–308.

Alpherts WCJ & Aldenkamp AP. Computerized neuropsychological assessment of cognitive functioning in children with epilepsy. *Epilepsia*, 1990(suppl. 4), 31:35–40.

Conners CK. A teacher rating scale for use in drug studies with children. *Am J Psychiatry*, 1969, 126:884–888.

Davidoff RA & Johnson LC. Paroxysmal EEG activity and cognitive motor performance. *EEG Clin Neurophysiol*, 1964, 16:343–354.

Kasteleijn-Nolst Trenité DGA, Bakker DJ, Binnie CD, Buerman A & van Raaij M. Psychological effects of subclinical epileptiform discharges: Scholastic skills. *Epilepsy Res*, 1988, 2:111–116.

Milner B. Interhemispheric differences in the localization of psychological processes in man. *British Medical Bulletin*, 1971, 27:272–277.

Prechtl HFR, Boeke PE & Schut T. The electroencephalogram and performance in epileptic patients. *Neurology*, 1961, 11:296–302.

Rugland AL. (1990). Subclinical epileptogenic activity. In: M Sillanpää, SI Johannsen, G Blennow & M Dam (eds.), *Paediatric epilepsy* (pp. 217–223). London: Wrightson Biomedical.

Rugland AL. Neuropsychological assessment of cognitive functioning in children with epilepsy. *Epilepsia*, 1990 (suppl. 4):42–44.

Rugland AL & Bjørnœs H. Systematic changes in attention as an effect of methylphenidate in children with epilepsy and serious attentional problems. European Brain and Behavior society, Workshop, 1987, Abstract.

Rugland AL & Bjørnœs H, Henriksen O & Løyning A. The development of computerized tests as a routine procedure in clinical EEG practice for the evaluation of cognitive changes in patients with epilepsy. 17th International Congress, 1987, Abstracts (p. 102).

Schwab RS. A method of measuring consciousness in petit mal epilepsy. *J Nerv Ment Dis*, 1939, 89:690-691.

Seidenberg M, Beck N, Geisser M, et al. Neuropsychological correlates of academic achievement of children with epilepsy. *J Epilepsy*, 1988, 1:23-29.

Siebelink BM, Bakker DJ, Binnie CD, et al. Psychological effects of sub-clinical epileptiform EEG discharges in children: General intelligence tests. *Epilepsy Res*, 1988, 2:117-121.

Sprague RL & Sleator EK. What is the proper dose of stimulant drugs in children? *J Abnorm Child Psychol*, 1975, 6(3):311, 324.

Tizard B & Margerison JH. Psychological functions during wave-spike discharge. *Br J Soc Clin Psychol*, 1963a, 3:6-15.

Tizard B & Margerison JH. The relationship between generalized paroxysmal EEG discharges and various test situations in 2 epileptic patients. *J Neurol Neurosurg Psychiat*, 1963b, 26:308-313.

8

Methods of Detecting Transitory Cognitive Impairment During Epileptiform EEG Discharges

C.D. Binnie
Maudsley Hospital
London, England

Introduction

Among the earliest findings of clinical electroencephalography was the occurrence of discharges of spikes or spikes and slow waves during epileptic seizures. However, it rapidly emerged that the relationship between such EEG phenomena and clinical ictal events was complex: Many discharges were subclinical, occurring without evident behavioral change (Gibbs et al. 1936; Lennox 1941); yet, by contrast, many apparently subclinical discharges were themselves accompanied by subtle cognitive changes, detectable by psychological testing. Thus Schwab (1939), using a simple reaction time task, demonstrated that during spike-and-wave activity, even in the absence of an overt seizure, there was often a decrement in performance, as evidenced by increased reaction time or total failure to respond. Some 40 subsequent studies have confirmed the occurrence of such brief cognitive deficits during subclinical discharges, called Transitory Cognitive Impairment (TCI) by Binnie (1980).

TCI calls into question the concept of an epileptic seizure as an overt clinical phenomenon rather than an electrophysiological finding: Arguably a brief cognitive change accompanying an epileptiform discharge meets current definitions of a seizure, in which case the accompanying EEG activity cannot properly be termed, subclinical or interictal. Of more practical consequence is the contribution, if any, of TCI to the cognitive deficits that hinder the psychosocial functioning of many persons with epilepsy. Some authors have adopted the view that generalized spike-and-wave activity is always accompanied by some cognitive impairment (Kooi & Hovey 1957; Delgado-Escueta 1979). Few, however, would consider it reasonable to base clinical action on such an assumption, for instance by attempting to suppress the discharges with medication, without evidence that TCI is occurring and likely to cause a significant deficit of psychosocial function.

As a preliminary to the study of TCI, both in the clinical assessment of the individual patient, and in order to address the wider issue of its general importance as a source of disability, it was necessary to develop psychological tests suitable for demonstrating TCI during EEG examination. This has proved less simple than might be expected.

Effect of Discharge Type

There is general agreement that TCI is most readily demonstrable during 3 c/sec, well organized, high voltage, generalized spike-wave activity, and that impairment is less likely to be found the more the discharge differs from the classical pattern seen in absence epilepsy (Kooi & Hovey 1957; Mirsky & Van Buren 1965; Browne et al. 1974; Hutt et al. 1977b; Davidov & Johnson 1964; Goode et al. 1970). Until recently, studies of the effects of focal discharges were few and nonrigorous: Some purported to show TCI during focal epileptiform activity (Kooi & Hovey 1957), others did not (Prechtl et al. 1961; Mirsky 1960).

The probability of finding TCI is also related to the length of the discharges, the duration of generalized spike-and-wave activity required for consistent demonstration of impairment being variously estimated as 3 s to over 8 s (Tizard & Margerison 1963; Mirsky & Van Buren 1965; Schwab 1941; Davidov & Johnson 1964; Goode et al. 1970). Browne et al. (1974) detected no effect of discharge length.

It is clear that the detectability of TCI depends on the task used, some tests being more sensitive than others, and some showing selective effects of particular discharge types. Thus more recent investigations, using more sensitive test methods, have shown an incidence of TCI during focal discharges no less than that accompanying generalized spike-and-wave activity, and have found the type of cognitive impairment to be specific to the side of the focus (Aarts et al. 1984; Shewmon & Erwin 1988).

Tests Used for Detection of TCI

Simple Reaction Time

Simple reaction time (RT) is increased in many subjects with sustained generalized bursts of spike-and-wave activity, but not during every discharge

(Browne et al. 1974; Chatrian et al. 1970; Porter et al. 1973; Schwab 1941; Yeager & Guerrant 1957; Grisell et al. 1964; Tuvo 1958). Tizard and Margerison (1963) found a response to a majority of stimuli even during overt absences but did not cite RTs, which Browne et al. (1974) found to be prolonged in 65% of discharges. The sensory modality does not appear to affect the findings.

Choice Reaction Time

Variable results are reported for choice RTs, but most authors find these to be more sensitive to disruption by TCI than are simple RTs. Prechtl et al. (1961) detected no effect of epileptiform activity whereas increased choice RTs and errors were observed by Tizard and Margerison (1963) in all subjects. Lehmann (1963) observed TCI during spike-wave activity but, uniquely, found shorter RTs and reduced errors in the second preceding the discharge. Hutt et al. (1977b) demonstrated a linear relationship between RT and the information transmitted by each stimulus (log to base 2 of the number of possible equiprobable stimuli), and found that the regression coefficient was increased during discharges; that is, the rate of transmission of information was reduced.

Signal Detection Tasks

Tizard and Margerison (1963) obtained somewhat inconsistent results using an auditory digit detection task. The continuous performance task of Mirsky and Van Buren (1965) showed the incidence of demonstrable TCI varied between subjects and across sessions from 100% to zero. Hutt (1972) similarly demonstrated that TCI was more often found as the rate of gain of information increased. Hutt et al. (1977a) also employed an auditory detection task and found, surprisingly, no elevation in threshold but that the subjects employed a more conservative decision criterion during discharges.

Simple Motor Tasks

Several authors have employed simple motor tasks, such as tapping, key pressing, or string pulling (Mirsky & Van Buren 1965; Chatrian et al. 1970; Yeager & Guerrant 1957; Shimazono et al. 1953; Hauser 1960; Davidov & Johnson 1964). These are relatively insensitive to the effects of TCI, as indeed are simple motor tasks with a greater cognitive component, such as the use of a pursuit-rotor (Goode et al. 1970) and the drawing test of Guey et al. (1965). Any effects appear to be delayed, appearing only gradually 2 s or 3 s after onset of a prolonged discharge.

Tests of Attention and Recall

Various forms of digit retention tests have been used (Hutt 1972; Davidov & Johnson 1964; Geller & Geller 1970), with differing conclusions as to their sensitivity. Serial-sevens, counting backward, mental arithmetic, and finger counting have been employed, and also answering questions concerning written material (Shimazono et al. 1953; Davidov & Johnson 1964; Jus & Jus 1962; Ishihara & Yoshii 1967). TCI was found in about one-third of discharges and in two-thirds of patients. Retrograde amnesia has also been demonstrated. The delayed identification test of Mirsky and Van Buren (1965) showed a variable effect of discharges between stimulus and recall (5.0% to 54.5% errors) but was more sensitive to discharges occurring during the stimulus. Similarly, Aarts et al. (1984) using a short-term memory task, found effects of TCI only when the discharges fell during presentation of the material to be recalled, but no disruption by discharges during the response. Milstein and Stevens (1961), by contrast, found no effect on verbal learning or on conditioned avoidance.

General Tests of Intelligence

Various subtests of the Wechsler and the Halstead Battery have been used. Chatrian et al. (1970) found no effect but Kooi and Hovey (1957) "never obtained an adequate solution to a problem" during generalized spike-wave activity. Siebelink et al. (1988) showed selective effects of TCI on different subtests of a general children's intelligence test, and suggested this might contribute to the abnormal subtest profiles exhibited by many patients with epilepsy.

Ad Hoc Clinical Tests

In clinical practice, useful information may be obtained by informal tests, such as checking whether or not the patient reacts to his or her name, continues reading aloud, or answers questions (Tizard & Margerison 1963; Shimazono et al. 1953; Jus & Jus 1962; Goldie & Green 1961; Bates 1953). Language function appears especially sensitive to TCI.

Real-Life Tasks

Using EEG telemetry during performance of real-life tasks, Kasteleijn-Nolst Trenité et al. (1987, 1988) have demonstrated disruptive effects of subclinical discharges on practical skills: reading, and driving a car.

The Nature of Psychological Deficit During TCI

A consideration in design of tests suitable for detecting TCI is the nature of the cognitive deficit. This was neglected by many of the earlier investigators, who apparently regarded the effect as being a nonspecific impairment of attention requiring no further analysis. However, Tizard and Margerison (1963) explained the differing sensitivities of various tests to TCI in terms of reduced channel capacity. Hutt (1972) and colleagues (1977a,b), in a series of elegant studies attempted a more detailed analysis of the cognitive defects and indeed obtained clear evidence that a reduced rate of information transmission is one of the features of TCI. However, they also demonstrated an adaptive response to the impairment produced by spike-wave activity—namely, an elevation of the decision criterion in a signal detection task (Hutt et al. 1977a). A short-term memory disturbance is often an important feature of the deficit and, when the stimulus consists of sequentially presented material as in a digit retention task, recall of the last elements is most disturbed (Hutt & Gilbert 1980). Recent studies of the effects of focal discharges (Aarts et al. 1984; Shewmon & Erwin 1988) suggest cognitive effects of discharges to be much more discrete than previously thought and determined by the side (right or left) of discharge. The finding of material-specific deficits implies a need for a battery of tests to screen for TCI because this may take different forms in different subjects.

Considerations in the Design of Tasks for Detecting TCI

An important practical consideration in the design of a test for investigating TCI is the difficulty of capturing sufficient discharges during performance of the task. During testing in the alert, eyes-open state which is obviously of most practical relevance, discharges in most patients are brief and few, and are in any event suppressed by attending to the task. Most research studies concern selected patients with exceptionally high rates of discharge, and then often have to resort to group statistics in order to show any significant effects. If one wishes to detect TCI and assess its possible psychosocial consequences as a clinical service in any individual patient who exhibits subclinical discharges, the tests require a more general applicability than those previously used in research.

The chances of capturing sufficient discharges to establish any effect on cognition will be increased if the task requires continuous cognitive performance and is sufficiently agreeable for the subject to be willing to work at it for a considerable period of time. It has been suggested (Porter et al. 1973; Binnie & Lloyd 1973) that a discontinuous task, such as reaction time, would be acceptable if the presentation of stimuli could be triggered by the discharges. However, this has the drawback that a finite length of discharge is required for the recognition algorithm, delivery of test stimuli before the end of a very brief discharge is therefore impossible. More important is the theoretical objection that discharge probability is affected by state of awareness so that discharges may occur preferentially when the patient is already inattentive. Although any claims for the demonstration of TCI are open to this criticism, the problems are less if testing is continuous and performance during a discharge can be compared with that immediately preceding or following it. Obviously, the task should suppress discharges as little as possible; although the effects of arousal on epileptiform activity are variable, most subjects will show the highest discharge rate if the task is neither stressful nor tedious. It is apparent from the literature reviewed above that too-easy tasks are likely to be insensitive to effects of TCI. As the subjects needing to be tested cover a range of ages and abilities, an ideal task will be adaptive to the performance level of the individual patient. Finally, recent observations on laterality or material-specific effects of TCI suggest that tests should be designed to assess different cognitive functions and to detect neuropsychological deficits reflecting disturbances of different brain regions.

Practical Tests for TCI

A task has been developed (Aarts et al. 1984) that may meet, to a considerable degree, the criteria set out above. This is a short-term memory test presented in the form of a computer game and bearing some resemblance to Corsi's Block Tapping Test. An array of blocks is presented on the screen; some of these flash on and off in a sequence, which the subject is asked to reproduce immediately by pointing at the blocks with a light pen. A similar task employs verbal material comprising a sequence of four-letter words on the screen, which the subject is then required to point out in sequence from a list. In a recently revised version, we have substituted numbers for words, in order to reduce the possibility of using nonverbal imagery, but the numeric and verbal variants give very similar results. The tasks are adaptive, the difficulty (sequence length) being adjusted automatically on the basis of results, such that the subject responds correctly to 50% of trials. The tasks are made more entertaining by the use of color and sound effects and most subjects above a mental age of 6 years are able and willing to work at them for periods of up to 1 h. Over this prolonged period of testing there is usually rapid habituation of any initial suppression of discharges by the task and in the series studied by Aarts et al. (1984) it was possible to capture sufficient discharges to draw some conclusions about the presence of TCI in 90% of cases.

In order to relate performance to the occurrence of discharges the task is regarded as a series of trials, each commencing with a warning tone, 1 s before the start of the flashing blocks sequence and terminating at the end of the response, either completion of the sequence, commission of a response error or hesitation without use of the light pen for a preset period (usually 8 s). Results are analyzed by simple tests of association between correct and incorrect response and occurrence, or nonoccurrence, of a discharge during the trial in question. More detailed analyses address effects of discharges at particular stages of the trial sequence (pretrial period, stimulus presentation, stimulus-response interval, response), and of different types of epileptiform activity. To facilitate assessment of the timing of discharges, the task is monitored on the polygraph used to record the EEG. A special-purpose character generator is driven (by print commands) through the serial RS232 port of the computer, annotating the chart with trial numbers and elapsed time (for synchronization with a video/EEG-telemetry system). A DA converter card is used to output pulses to the chart that indicates the timing of stimuli and responses. It can also output time and trial numbers as BCD codes, for use without the special character generator. To provide further independence of specific hardware, a cursor controlled by the computer keyboard can be substituted for the light pen. A second channel of the DA converter may be used to trigger an electrical stimulator to induce discharges at selected sites in patients with intracranial electrodes. Because such patients may have large numbers of spontaneous discharges, it is sometimes difficult to capture sufficient numbers of discharge-free trials; the stimulus probability is therefore adjustable to a level at which it is anticipated that an adequate number of trials will be free of either spontaneous or induced discharges.

The progress of the task is logged on the computer's hard disk: trial number, time of day, electrical stimulation (if used), sequence length, correct or incorrect response, and reaction time being recorded for each trial. An interactive program facilitates entry and editing of information regarding discharge type, duration, and timing, so that these can be collated with trial results. A further program tests for significance of any association between discharge occurrence and error, and allows various filters to be applied (to determine effects of discharges of a particular type or occurring at a particular point in the stimulus-response sequence). All programs are available as GW or Quick-BASIC and run on an IBM AT or compatible, with an EGA or VGA monitor.

During the original evaluation study by Aarts et al. (1984) video monitoring was used throughout testing, and any patients showing overt seizures during the investigation were excluded. It was found that the application of this criterion virtually eliminated any subjects with generalized symmetrical spike-wave activity of more than 3 s duration as these invariably exhibited clinical signs, during some or all discharges. Despite the exclusion of just those subjects who, according to the literature, were most likely to exhibit TCI, an effect statistically significant within each individual was found in 50% of those considered testable. Indeed, the sensitivity of the tasks was sufficient to demonstrate TCI not only in the presence of generalized discharges, but with equal frequency during asymmetrical or focal discharges. Effects of focal discharges were modality-specific, TCI being more readily demonstrable in association with right-sided discharges using the blocks task, and with left-sided discharges using the verbal version of the test.

Test Evaluation and Conclusions

An evaluation study of the tests described suggested that these were suitable for routine use in clinical practice (Aarts et al. 1984). Of 46 subjects with frequent interictal discharges in the eyes-open alert state, two were eliminated because of overt myoclonic seizures, apparently induced by the task; another showed an increase in epileptiform activity so marked that he became untestable, as discharges occurred on all trials. Twelve showed a decrease in discharge rate, but in only 4 was this of such a degree as to render testing impracticable. The tasks were well tolerated by patients of average intelligence 8 years of age and older, who would often work continuously for up to an hour trying to improve their performance.

TCI was demonstrated in more than 50% of subjects. Interestingly, there were material-specific effects of lateralized discharges, those on the left being more often accompanied by performance decrement on the verbal task, those on the right with impairment on the blocks test.

The effect of laterality of discharges has been confirmed using the same and similar tasks by Rugland (this volume) and for simple reaction times to left- and right-sided visual stimuli by Shewmon and Erwin (1988). These findings imply that TCI is not due merely to a global attention deficit, but that the impairment may be specific to cognitive functions thought to be lateralized, and possibly localized, close to the site of abnormal discharge. This has interesting wider implications for neuropsychological testing in epilepsy. Any cognitive deficits found, apart from those due to medication, are generally assumed to be static, most probably the result of cerebral pathology, and irremediable. If episodic cerebral dysfunction contributes both to general and to material-specific deficits, there may be some difficulty in interpreting psychological findings after treatment. For instance, an absence of cognitive deterioration, or indeed an apparent improvement, following surgery or administration of an experimental antiepileptic drug, may in part reflect a reduction of TCI due to suppression of interictal discharges.

The possible psychosocial disabilities resulting from TCI remain uncertain, as does the possibility of their relief by measures intended to reduce the causative discharges. Some patients do demonstrably experience social problems because of TCI (Aarts et al. 1984), and some have benefited from suppression of discharges by medication. The extent of the problem remains unknown and, in view of the adverse cognitive effects of antiepileptic medication, and the difficulty of suppressing EEG discharges by drugs, further studies are clearly required to determine criteria for therapeutic intervention in patients with TCI.

References

Aarts JHP, Binnie CD, Smit AM & Wilkins AJ. Selective cognitive impairment during focal and generalised epileptiform EEG activity. *Brain*, 1984, 107:293-308.

Bates JAV. A technique for identifying changes in consciousness. *Electroencephalogr. Clin. Neurophysiol.*, 1953, 5:445-446.

Binnie CD. (1980). Detection of transitory cognitive impairment during epileptiform

EEG discharges: Problems in clinical practice. In: BM Kulig, H Meinardi & G Stores (eds.), *Epilepsy and behaviour '79* (pp 91-97). Lisse: Swets and Zeitlinger.

Binnie CD & Lloyd DSL. A technique for measuring reaction times during paroxysmal discharges. *Electroencephalogr. Clin. Neurophysiol.*, 1973, 35:418.

Browne TR, Penry SK, Porter RS & Dreifuss F. Responsiveness before, during and after spike-wave paroxysms. *Neurology (Minneap.)*, 1974, 24:659-665.

Chatrian GE, Lettich E, Miller LH, Green JR & Kupfer C. Pattern-sensitive epilepsy. Part 2: Clinical changes, tests of responsiveness and motor output, alterations of evoked potentials and therapeutic measures. *Epilepsia*, 1970, 11:151-162.

Davidov RA & Johnson LC. Paroxysmal EEG activity and cognitive motor performance. *Electroencephalogr. Clin. Neurophysiol.*, 1964, 16:343-354.

Delgado-Escueta AV. Epileptogenic paroxysms: Modern approaches and clinical correlations. *Neurology (Minneap.)*, 1979, 29:1014-1022.

Geller MR & Geller A. Brief amnestic effects of spike-wave discharges. *Neurology (Minneap.)*, 1970, 20:380-381.

Gibbs FA, Lennox WG & Gibbs EL. The electroencephalogram in diagnosis and in localization of epileptic seizures. *Arch. Neurol. Psychiatry*, 1936, 36:1225-1235.

Goldie L & Green JM. Spike and wave discharges and alterations of conscious awareness. *Nature (London)*, 1961, 191:200-201.

Goode DJ, Penry JK & Dreifuss FE. Effects of paroxysmal spike-wave and continuous visual motor performance. *Epilepsia*, 1970, 11:241-254.

Grisell JL, Levin SM, Cohen BD & Rodin EA. Effects of subclinical seizure activity on overt behavior. *Neurology (Minneap.)*, 1964, 14:133-135.

Guey J, Tassinari CA, Charles C & Coquery C. Variations du niveau d'efficience en relation avec des décharges épileptiques paroxystiques. *Rev. Neurol. (Paris)*, 1965, 112:311-317.

Hauser F. (1960). *Perception et responses motrices au cours des paroxysmes de pointes-ondes*. Paris: Foulon.

Hutt SJ. Experimental analysis of brain activity and behaviour in children with 'minor' seizures. *Epilepsia*, 1972, 13:520-534.

Hutt SJ & Gilbert S. Effects of evoked spike-wave discharges upon short-term memory in patients with epilepsy. *Cortex*, 1980, 16:445-457.

Hutt, SJ, Denner S & Newton J. Auditory thresholds during evoked spike-wave activity in epileptic patients. *Cortex*, 1977a, 12:249-257.

Hutt SJ, Newton S & Fairweather H. Choice reaction time and EEG activity in children with epilepsy. *Neuropsychologica*, 1977b, 5:257-267.

Ishihara T & Yoshii N. The interaction between paroxysmal EEG activities and continuous addition work of Uchida-Kraepelin psychodiagnostic test. *Med. J. Osaka Univ.*, 1967, 18:75-85.

Jus A & Jus K. Retrograde amnesia in petit mal. *Arch. Gen. Psychiatry*, 1962, 6:163-167.

Kasteleijn-Nolst Trenité DGA, Bakker DJ, Binnie CD, Buerman A & van Raaij M. Psychological effects of subclinical epileptiform discharges: Scholastic skills. *Epilepsy Research*, 1988, 2:111-116.

Kasteleijn-Nolst Trenité DGA, Riemersma JBJ, Binnie CD, Smit AM & Meinardi H. The influence of subclinical epileptiform EEG discharges on driving behaviour. *Electroencephalogr. Clin. Neurophysiol.*, 1987, 67:167-170.

Kooi KA & Hovey HB. Alterations in mental function and paroxysmal cerebral activity. *Arch. Neurol. Psychiatry*, 1957, 78:264-271.

Lehmann HJ. Präparoxysmale Weckreakton bei pyknoleptischen Absencen. *Arch. Psychiatr. Nervenkr.*, 1963, 204:417-426.

Lennox WG. Cited by Schwab (see Schwab 1941).

Milstein V & Stevens JR. Verbal and conditioned avoidance learning during abnormal EEG discharge. *J. Nerv. Ment. Dis.*, 1961, 132:50-60.

Mirsky AF. The relationship between paroxysmal EEG activity and performance on a vigilance task in epileptic patients. *A. Psychol.*, 1960, 15:486.

Mirsky AF & Van Buren HM. On the nature of the "absence" in centrencephalic epilepsy: A study of some behavioural electroencephalographic and autonomic factors. *Electroencephalogr. Clin. Neurophysiol.*, 1965, 18:334-338.

Porter RJ, Penry SK & Dreifuss FE. Responsiveness at the onset of spike-wave bursts. *Electroencephalogr. Clin. Neurophysiol.*, 1973, 34:239-245.

Prechtl HFR, Boeke PE & Schut T. The electroencephalogram and performance in epileptic patients. *Neurology (Minneap.)*, 1961, 11:296-302.

Schwab RS. A method of measuring consciousness in petit-mal epilepsy. *J. Nerv. Ment. Dis.*, 1939, 89:690-691.

Schwab RS. The influence of visual and auditory stimuli on electroencephalographic tracing of petit-mal. *Am. J. Psychiatry*, 1941, 97:1301-1312.

Shewmon DA & Erwin RJ. The effect of focal interictal spikes on perception and reaction time. II: Neuroanatomic specificity. *Electroencephalogr. Clin. Neurophysiol.*, 1988, 69:338-352.

Shimazono Y, Hirai T, Okuma T, Fukuda T & Yamamasu E. Disturbance of consciousness in petit mal epilepsy. *Epilepsia*, 1953, 2:49-55.

Siebelink BM, Bakker DJ, Binnie CD & Kasteleijn-Nolst Trenité DGA. Psychological effects of sub-clinical epileptiform EEG discharges in children: General intelligence tests. *Epilepsy Research*, 1988, 2:117-121.

Tizard B & Margerison JH. Psychological functions during wave-spike discharges. *Br. J. Soc. Clin. Psychol.*, 1963, 3:6-15.

Tuvo F. Contribution a l'etude des niveaux de conscience au cours des paroxysmes epileptiques infracliniques. *Electroencephalogr. Clin. Neurophysiol.*, 1958, 10: 715-718.

Yeager CL & Guerrant JS. Subclinical epileptic seizures. *Calif. Med.*, 1957, 86:242-247.

9

Statistical Issues in the Computerized Assessment of Cognitive Function

Tony Johnson
Medical Research Council Biostatistics Unit
Cambridge, United Kingdom

Introduction

The past 15 years have seen the publication of a flurry of books devoted to the randomized clinical trial (RCT) (Good 1976; Johnson & Johnson 1977; Boissel & Klimt 1979; Schwartz et al. 1980; Tygstrup et al. 1982; Shapiro & Louis 1983; Pocock 1983; Buyse et al. 1984; Friedman et al. 1985; Spriet & Simon 1985; Meinert 1986; Rotmensz et al. 1989; Jones & Kenward 1989). These texts describe the general principles of trial design and organization, and contain much sound and sensible advice regarding their conduct and analysis. However, the nature and requirements of RCTs varies from one medical specialty to another, and there are good reasons for textbooks devoted to clinical trials within specific subdisciplines of medicine. Such books require extensive collaboration between physicians and statisticians, and represent a challenge which thus far has only been partially met within cancer (Buyse et al. 1984; Rotmensz et al. 1989), much less so in other areas. The first text devoted to RCTs in neurology has recently appeared (Capildeo & Orgogozo 1988).

There is a need for further refinement—not only to specific diseases such as epilepsy, but (as this workshop has shown) to specific issues: The computerized assessment of cognitive function in patients with epilepsy, for example. The purpose of this chapter is to discuss generally some of the important statistical issues of RCTs, and specifically within the context of computerized testing of patients maintained on antiepileptic drugs, where the main interest lies in assessment of the comparative effects of the drugs. It is now widely appreciated that the RCT is the only type of study that can provide unbiased estimates of such effects. Inevitably some of the remarks will also apply to epidemiological studies where the main focus is assessment of the level of risk, and those factors which influence it.

The issues will be discussed and illustrated against the background and experience of an open randomized clinical trial designed to compare the efficacy of four antiepileptic drugs (carbamazepine, phenobarbitone, phenytoin, and sodium valproate) to control seizures in patients with epilepsy. This trial was conducted in two main centers, London (Department of Neurology, King's College Hospital and Department of Paediatric Neurology, Guy's Hospital) and Department of Neurosciences, Walton Hospital, Liverpool. Between 1981 and 1987, 174 children and 243 adults were recruited. Patients randomized from the two hospitals in London were also scheduled for IQ assessment and computerized testing of specific cognitive functions.

Computer Optimism

Since the introduction of electronic computing machines in the late 1940s, there has been revolutionary changes in central processing units (CPUs) speed and capacity to store, retrieve, and transfer information. The speed of the fastest machines today—over 3000 megaflops or million floating-point operations per second (Corcoran 1991)—dwarfs some aspects of the mental processing power of the human brain. Indeed we have moved full circle in that these machines are now used to assess the mental functioning and capacity of the race which invented them. We must remember, however, that computers are still no better than the programs that drive them. Although computers offer an opportunity for better standardization in the testing environment as well as the facility for more precise measurement of response, they do not enhance the content and validity of the test instruments themselves. Today, practical applications include: storing questionnares in memory; programs that check and cross-check responses for relevance and consistency, and that sequence questions and tasks in a logical order with appropriate skips to avoid interrogation for irrelevant information. The computer neither disputes a basic questionnaire or task design (though it may help to structure it), nor does it query the validity of the information stored, and it definitely does not automatically guarantee a better form of test. It is worthwhile remembering that the development of tests of cognitive function requires considerable skill, combined with extensive testing and validation. Those tests that are developed for computer assessment require full collaboration between computer scientists and programmers and need extensive checking—especially if interfacing with various computers. Also, self-checking programs are necessary in order to ensure that the tests are working properly to some minimal standard. Where different forms (manual and computerized) of a test exist they should be compared, and it should never optimistically be assumed that the computerized form is always the better! Computers offer many opportunities for subtle changes to test procedures, and several versions of one test may be available; these should be compared using statistical analyses appropriate to method comparison studies, not correlation coefficients (Altman & Bland 1983; Bland & Altman 1986; Chinn 1990).

Missing Data

It may appear somewhat perverse to concentrate near the beginning on data that are "missing" rather than those which are available for analysis. However, in biomedical studies, it is missing data that cause the most serious difficulties. While they do not surface as a problem until the stage of analysis, missing data are a consequence of poor study design, and it is here that they must be anticipated and minimized. In addition, methods for coping with them in the analysis should be decided.

The major sources of missing data in RCTs of antiepileptic drugs where the aim is to assess comparative efficacy as well as effects on cognitive function are summarized in Table 1. The most common source derives from the failure of outpatients to attend hospital clinics. In RCTs of this type patients will be scheduled for follow-up for at least 2 years and perhaps for much longer. Attenuation of the sample by loss to follow-up will cause more problems for the analysis of computerized assessments than for the measures of efficacy because, although far from ideal, information about seizure recurrence and drug side effects may be obtained from general practitioner' records or by direct contact with patients (for example, by telephone). Retrospective information about missed computerized assessments cannot be obtained.

TABLE 1

Major Sources of Missing Data in Clinical Trials with
Computerized Tests of Cognitive Function

1. Patient nonattendance	
2. Patient attends but is	
• too young	• unable to spare time
• too elderly	• unable to cope with computers
• physically handicapped	• unable to understand test instructions
• mentally handicapped	• unable to complete test—too difficult
3. Computer malfunction	

There are several strategies that help to reduce the volume of missing data arising from patient nonattendance. The schedule of follow-up visits may be simplified to attempt computerized assessment at intervals of not less than 1 year, or even longer. Focusing attention on just an initial assessment at study entry, and a final one after a set interval is sufficient to provide broad comparison of longer-term effects of antiepileptic drugs. The exclusion of interim assessments will sacrifice information about the emergence of differential drug effects. However, for the purpose of analysis and the drawing of reasoned and substantiated conclusions, it is better to have almost complete information about one or two points in time, than a patchwork of data from an over-ambitious testing schedule. And in many RCTs the schedule of testing is far too elaborate, as evidenced by the volume of missing data. The best solution to this problem and one that can be readily implemented following the development of transportable PCs is an arrangement to visit the patient at home. Disturbances in the test environment may be avoided by using "walk-in" vans. The introduction of laptop machines will ultimately make transportation much easier, but at present they lack the sophisticated graphics and displays necessary for computerized tests. Restriction of testing to "captive" populations, such as hospital inpatients, does not help here. First, because such patients are not representative of the majority of patients prescribed antiepileptic drugs in the community; and second, because patients who are hospitalized over long periods may be unsuitable for computerized testing. Captive populations may be used in the early stages of drug development and testing although not for the detection of anything other than extreme effects on cognitive function.

Another series of problems arises when patients are available for assessment but cannot cope with computerized tests. An obvious example is the very young child who cannot physically depress computer keys, as well as slightly older ones who do not comprehend the structure of computerized tests sufficiently to execute them. Reading ability is obviously essential for tests where instructions must be read from the terminal. The infirmities of old age—especially poor eyesight, deafness, rheumatism, lack of mobility, and dementia—produce difficulties in the elderly. Physical handicaps, such as blindness and restricted movement, are sufficient to exclude subjects from computerized tests, but mental handicaps may not be. Some subjects with mental handicaps are well able to understand the requirements of some tests, even though they may exhibit much slower response times than comparable subjects who are not handicapped (Simpson et al. 1991).

There are, however, more subtle examples of patients who though apparently normal, cannot cope with the computer testing environment. Faced with a keyboard and terminal they may stare blankly at it, and appear unable to respond to the given stimuli. There have been many guidelines, full of sound advice about the need for soft lighting, adjustable seating, well-designed keyboards, tilting screens, distracting backdrops, and so on, for employees engaged in extended use of computers (Health and Safety Executive 1983, 1986). Some of these suggestions are useful with computerized tests, and their application may help reduce patients' reluctance or anxiety when faced with an inanimate screen. I suggest that the computer environment should be tidy (without tangles of computer cables or trailing wires), the software should be produced to commercial standards with full use of colors and graphics, and must be user-friendly; there should be no display of unnecessary information (particularly computer codes) and certainly no fiddling with plugs, switches, or cables in front of patients to get machines to work properly. When feasible, keyboards should be simplified with keys sufficient for the battery of assessments and no more. There is no need to confront any patient with the full 102-key IBM standard keyboard! Computer equipment peripheral to the test should be out of sight.

The discussion above has focused on subjects unable to engage in any or most computerized tests. While it is not essential that every patient entered in a RCT of antiepileptic drugs should undergo computerized testing (adequate power may be achievable for such tests without this guarantee; see the discussion under "Sample Size"), we do need to ensure that the assessments used are suitable for the majority of patients. And, in addition, we need sufficient knowledge of the chosen assessments themselves to be clear which subjects are requested to undergo this type of testing, and which are not. The trial protocol should be clear about entry criteria to the trial itself, and also about the characteristics of patients excluded from certain forms of testing.

Other problems occur because of missing information. In studies that use a battery of tests of varying complexity some subjects will be able to complete the simpler but not the more complicated tests. For example, with tests assessing reaction times (Simple Reaction Time, Choice Reaction Time, SAUL) (Sternberg 1966), most subjects will be able to complete the first two, fewer will complete the last. The SAUL in particular has a complex structure with a series of 1, 3, or 5 digits followed by a single-probe digit flashed on-screen nearly every second; the subject is required to indicate—using two different keys—whether or not the probe digit was included in the series. Some subjects are able to respond to the shorter series but cannot cope with the longer. The changing patterns of missing information frustrate any simple analysis. It is unclear how to deal with data from patients who complete one test but not another, and even less clear how to handle data from partially completed tests, especially if the full structure of the test is to be incorporated in the analysis. Analysis of available data from each test will result in sample changes from one set of results to another, restriction to the set of patients who provide complete information on all tests can lead to the elimination of virtually the whole sample, and more important neither method can claim an unbiased comparison of treatments. The only feasible analysis may be one that examines the differing patterns of missing information!

In some studies, and especially those which include children, subjects who cannot undergo computerized tests at the initial, and perhaps some subsequent visits, will eventually be able to complete such tests, and perhaps provide complete information during later visits. These subjects pose just as many problems for analysis as those who provide initial assessments and then drop out. Observations missing at the onset of a study eliminate subjects from analysis of change, and do not allow adjustment using "baseline" information (analysis of covariance). Sound practical advice is to exclude from studies subjects who cannot provide important baseline information, and particularly in RCTs with multiple endpoints, stratify patients by whether or not they will participate in computerized assessments.

Recently there have been major developments in the techniques for analysis of longitudinal or follow-up data (Workshop on Methods for Longitudinal Data Analysis in Epidemiological and Clinical Studies 1988), and in their incorporation in standard computer packages (for example, the program BMDP5V in the BMDP suite) (Dixon 1988). These techniques essentially provide a statistical framework for modeling missing information, but not without some fairly stringent assumptions about the distribution of missing values, in particular the assumption that what is "missing" is unassociated with specific treatment ("missing at random").

Analysis of a complete dataset usually causes few problems, with just a few missing values we can usually find some sort of reasonable "fix-up," but with extensive missing data there are always problems, and the best solution is to adopt a design that minimizes these as far as possible.

Finally, a decade ago computers were less reliable than today, and it was not unusual to find patients who were keen to undergo computer assessment, and willingly sat in front of machines that on occasion, refused to work. Today that picture has changed, but routine maintenance and checking, together with back-up of programs, diskettes, and machines, may save some embarrassments!

Test Selection

There are several aspects of cognitive function that can now be assessed by computerized tests. These include reaction times, information processing, reasoning and decision making, as well as short- and long-term (verbal and nonverbal) memory. Additionally there is a variety of tests to assess each of these aspects. In any particular study several tests may be combined into a single battery to provide a comprehensive cognitive profile. A major requirement for any battery is that the majority of study participants should be able to complete the battery within a reasonable time, and that the tests included can be justified as scientifically necessary. Tests should not be included just because they happen to be available, or because they might be interesting. A test battery that extends over a period exceeding 30 min may induce fatigue or boredom, and could seriously jeopardize future cooperation by persuading patients not to collaborate in further assessments. The basic aim should be simplicity with minimal burden to the study participants.

The completed battery should be user-friendly and, as far as possible, based on a dialog, not a monolog. Information feedback to the patient, and a friendly sign-off may enhance future cooperation.

The tests selected for a battery should assess a range of cognitive functions, and be as independent of each other as possible. There is no point in including two tests that exhibit very high correlation when essentially they are measuring the same thing. While it is difficult to justify general rules for the selection of tests, it may be useful to remember that correlation coefficients exceeding 0.7 (in absolute value) are equivalent to one test explaining more than 50% of the variation in another. This may serve as a useful point at which to pitch the boundary between inclusion and exclusion, or at least a point beyond which the inclusion of tests in a battery requires special justification.

The order of tests within a battery also needs care because performance on one test may be modified by the tests presented earlier. While this may not be of immediate importance within a comparative study where *differences* between treatments are the main outcome, it does have implications for comparison of test performances across studies or with external standards. There appears to have been little research on the construction of batteries of computerized assessments, and in particular any need for relaxing or distracting intervals between successive tests.

The choice between several tests measuring similar aspects of cognitive function may be made on criteria of simplicity, level of understanding, comparability with previous studies and/or measures of reliability and variation. Tests with lower variation are more sensitive in the sense that they require smaller sample sizes to detect a specified effect.

Speed and/or Accuracy?

It is important that the properties of psychometric and other tests employed for evaluation in RCTs should be well understood, and this means that we should have a clear idea of what they measure, the characteristics of patients for whom they may be used, and how they may be analyzed. The clinical trial is not a vehicle for development of new tests, or indeed for extensive refinements to existing ones, and the temptation to pursue "add-on" studies of this type must be suppressed.

Quite clearly for a test such as simple reaction time (SRT) with a stimulus (a digit appearing on the monitor screen) and response (the subject depressing a key), the main outcome of interest is the interval between the two; that is, the reaction time. However, if a subject hits keys randomly without waiting for a stimulus then the time to response is not a legitimate measure of reaction time.

More complicated versions of these tests pose more difficult problems: for example when a subject is asked to respond to the appearance of an odd or even digit using different keys, but to ignore any other character. Not only can we measure reaction times following the correct responses, we can also assess accuracy by the number of times a subject responds "correctly" to odd and even digits. One subject may elect to respond very quickly to almost every character, thus achieving a fast reaction time but with low accuracy; another may respond slower, giving a much longer reaction time but with perfect accuracy. The analysis may consider the two outcomes, reaction time and accuracy, quite separately, but this ignores the trade-off between the two. Reporting the correlation between the two may provide a crude measure of the extent to which they interrelate, but ideally we may want to think in terms of combining reaction time and accuracy into a single overall measure. This is a major problem that requires resolution at the stage of test development.

Summary Measures

With a computerized assessment of simple or choice reaction times (RTs) the subjects often get a few practice runs to familiarize themselves both with the computer and with the test. The measurement of RT will then proceed over a set number of repeated trials. The computer may not allow access to the individual RTs, but may instead store or printout some summary statistics, such as the average and standard deviation (SD). It is essential that when summary statistics are produced, they should be known to be appropriate, and along with measures of location and spread, they must include the number of trials on which the summary measures are based. The best solution is that the computer store and allow access to the full data.

As an example, we can consider RTs from 3 patients in our trial shown in Table 2. Means (M) and standard deviations have been read off computer output and are assumed to be estimated from 30 trials of each test. The output

TABLE 2

Reaction Times for 3 Children on 2 Computerized Tasks

	Simple Reaction Time (msec)		Choice Reaction Time (msec)			
			Target 1		Target 2	
Subject	Mean	SD	Mean	SD	Mean	SD
1	274	53	419	106	515	168
2	596	156	781	136	619	189
3	669	157	987	278	894	256

Note: SD = standard deviation.

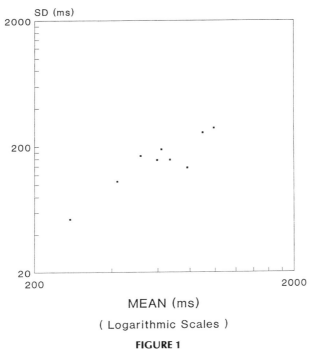

SD (ms)

MEAN (ms)

(Logarithmic Scales)

FIGURE 1

SD against Mean for Summary Statistics in Table 2 (ms = msec)

does not, but should, indicate the exact number of trials. We note that both the Ms and SDs for the choice RTs are larger than for the simple RTs, that there is a threefold variation in SDs and in addition it appears that the SDs increase with the Ms. These observations are sufficient to suggest that the underlying distributions of RTs may be positively skewed, and that Ms and SDs for RTs from the 30 trials are inappropriate summary statistics. If we plot the SDs against the Ms using logarithmic scales (as in Figure 1), then we see an approximate linear relationship between the two, indicating the need for data transformation to stabilize the variances. Of course in practice we would plot the data for the full sample, and for the two RTs separately, but Figure 1 is sufficient to illustrate the problem. The slope of the line is reasonably close to 1, and suggests that logarithmic transformation of the RTs from the individual trials is an adequate variance-stabilizing transformation. Ideally we would like to take logarithms of the individual RTs and then examine their distribution to see whether it is also approximately Normal. This we cannot do. Perhaps the best we can do is assume that RTs are approximately log-Normally distributed, and then estimate the parameters (μ and σ) of the underlying Normal distribution using the

Figure 2

If Reaction Times are log-Normally distributed with mean, M, and variance, V, then the underlying Normal distribution has mean, μ, and standard deviation, σ, where

$$\mu = \ln \left\{ \frac{M^2}{\sqrt{M^2 + V}} \right\}$$

$$\sigma^2 = \ln \left\{ \frac{V}{M^2} + 1 \right\}$$

FIGURE 2

formulae in Figure 2. We can then analyze the derived statistics in Table 3, and use these to estimate summary statistics including test statistics and confidence intervals, which depend on assumptions of Normality. Comparison of the back-transformed means in Table 3 with the means in Table 2 shows the correction produced by the transformation for the underlying skew. This example typifies the sort of rescue operation requested of statisticians after data collection, and which is best avoided.

A further example may be found in Wesnes et al. (1987) where the choice RTs (at the foot of their Table 2) exhibit a linear relationship between Ms and

TABLE 3

Mean and SD of the Normal Distributions Underlying the Data in Table 2*

Subject	Simple Reaction Time			Choice Reaction Time					
				Target 1			Target 2		
	Mean (μ)	SD (σ)	Back-transformed Mean (msec)	Mean (μ)	SD (σ)	Back-transformed Mean (msec)	Mean (μ)	SD (σ)	Back-transformed Mean (msec)
1	5.59	0.19	269	6.01	0.25	406	6.19	0.32	490
2	6.36	0.26	577	6.65	0.17	769	6.38	0.30	592
3	6.48	0.23	651	6.86	0.28	950	6.76	0.28	859

Note: *The means (μ) and SDs (σ) are calculated from the summary statistics in Table 2 using the formulae in Figure 2.

SDs (albeit over a narrow range of mean RTs). Here logarithmic transformation does not appear satisfactory, and the appropriate approach is far from clear. In both these examples we either need access to the raw data, namely the individual RTs, or we need sufficient basic knowledge of test performance to indicate the methods of analysis and appropriate summary statistics.

Reporting Tests and Batteries

Reports of studies that employ computerized assessments must include details of the individual tests and of the battery. The description of the battery itself should incorporate the order of test presentation, the pretest time and material (battery packaging), intertest times and material, and finally the sign-off. References (without details) may be given to batteries already published with full specifications, but any modification should be reported in full.

It is not sufficient to describe individual tests merely by title, unless a detailed specification already appears in print. Reference to a test of simple reaction time (SRT) is inadequate, and certainly does not facilitate comparison with other published studies. Computers allow many variations on the same test and it is informative to present exact details. For example, in the test of SRT in our trial, patients were required to depress a *single key* as soon as a *digit* appeared on the computer screen and the program ran until *35 responses* were obtained with a *random interval of between 1.0 and 3.5 s* between each digit; mean reaction time (and SD) were calculated from the *final 30* responses. Other tests of SRT are quite different, and the italicized text indicates the minimum specification. More complicated tests naturally require more detailed specification.

With the test of SRT described above we may ask: Why a digit (rather than a letter, a "space invader," or other animated character)? Why 35 responses? Why random intervals between 1.0 and 3.5s? and, Why use the final 30 responses? There are no satisfactory answers to these questions, though they certainly do need addressing. Indeed here is a great opportunity to employ some of the classical methods of experimentation to elicit the effects on reaction time of changes in these basic test characteristics. Some tests of SRT eliminate "outliers" prior to analysis (for example, very short RTs considered too rapid for human response), and very long RTs indicative of distraction. These strategies also require investigation especially with regard to within-patient (between-test) distribution.

Reporting Treatment Effects

In RCTs in epilepsy where there is prolonged patient follow-up, the randomized drug groups are sometimes compared using actuarial survival techniques (Peto et al. 1976, 1977), but with time to first seizure, time to achievement of 6 months' remission, or some other seizure-free period as the outcome of interest.

By contrast the tests of cognitive function are compared at predefined intervals, or perhaps just at the end of follow-up. Simple comparisons based on estimates of differences (sometimes ratios) between drug groups together with 95% confidence intervals (Altman et al. 1983; Gardner & Altman 1989) for these estimates are sensible and sufficient summary statistics; they are far superior to the mere reporting of P-values.

However, in RCTs, there is frequent concern that despite randomization, the individual drug groups may exhibit important differences in outcome as a result of some imbalance in the distributions of prognostic factors, for example, age, seizure type, or seizure history. Patients entered in RCTs are sometimes stratified prior to randomization (e.g., age < 16 years, age 16-60 years, age > 60 years) in an attempt to ensure that drug groups are roughly balanced on recognized prognostic factors. Stratification prior to randomization, however, cannot sensibly be used for more than two or three separate factors. It is not unusual to find in reports of RCTs a multitude of statistical significance tests carried out on baseline variables to determine which exhibit imbalance between the different treatment groups. Tests that are not significant (NS) at the 5% level ($P > 0.05$) are then considered to exhibit no imbalance for the associated variables whereas those that are significant ($P < 0.05$) are brought into the analysis as covariates (analysis of covariance). The differences between drug groups are thus adjusted for these variables.

This strategy is not a rational one and cannot be recommended (Altman 1985). The use of statistical significance tests in this screening role is not efficient, and alternative ways of selecting factors for which differences between treatment groups should be adjusted are required. The best method is to decide at the stage of RCT design (well before the start of patient recruitment), which factors to adjust for, relying on knowledge gained from previous studies, or clinical experience. Adjustment of treatment differences for effects unrelated to outcome will have negligible effect. The nominated factors will be dependent on the entry (inclusion and exclusion) criteria of the RCT. A list drawn from clinical consensus would be useful for RCTs using computerized assessment; it would include age, age squared, sex, experience of video games, severity of epilepsy, and many others.

Explanatory or Pragmatic Clinical Trials

There have been major developments over the past 15 years in our understanding of both the role and the interpretation of results from RCTs (Peto et al. 1976, 1977). It is now agreed that the only comparison of treatment effects guaranteed to be unbiased, is one based on the analysis of all randomized patients, and this forms the basis of philosophy of analysis under "intention to treat." Patients who are lost to follow-up, or who cannot undertake the trial assessments cannot contribute much to any form of sensible analysis without an assumption that their missing observations are unassociated with randomized treatment. Anything more than a small proportion of missing data will jeopardize or at least cast doubt on, the interpretation of the trial results. As indicated above this is one issue that should be considered during trial design (see "Missing Data" discussion above).

Apart from patients with missing information, there will also be patients who deviate from the clinical trial protocol in the sense that they do not take drugs or follow the schedules of treatment as intended; they may decide to reduce, or sometimes stop them (some patients even increase them), or alternatively their treatment may be modified by physicians including the prescription of other medication or forms of treatment. Such patients must not automatically be excluded from analysis.

A "pragmatic" analysis using all available patient data (intention to treat) compares the *policy* of giving one treatment with the *policy* of giving another (Schwartz et al. 1980; Peto et al. 1976, 1977; Johnson 1984). A pragmatic analysis estimates the average relative benefit or harm for the treatments under comparison in the treatment of future patients. Such an analysis should appear first in the report of a RCT.

Quite often—especially in drug trials—investigators are interested in the specific or direct effects of the drugs themselves, and attempt to estimate these by an analysis which excludes any patient who deviates from the study design. Such "explanatory" (or "on-treatment") analyses are mainly of scientific interest, and should follow rather than precede an analysis based on intention to treat. Reports should indicate, for each randomized treatment group, the number of patients actually randomized, the number excluded from the initial pragmatic analysis (and why), the number included in the pragmatic analysis, and then the numbers excluded from and included in each subsequent explanatory analysis; reasons for exclusion must be clearly stated because these allow readers to assess the validity of the report's conclusions.

Sample Size

The number of patients to be entered in a RCT must be estimated and justified during design to ensure that the study can indeed reach meaningful and clinically useful conclusions. There are different ways of accomplishing this; for example, by fixing the width of the confidence interval for the treatment difference (Day 1988), or more usually by a power calculation. Tables to estimate sample sizes for clinical trials on the basis of a power calculation are readily available, and cover most of the types of data that are likely to be encountered (Machin & Campbell 1987). However, power calculations cannot be conducted in isolation; they require some knowledge of the form of the main responses to be analyzed, the statistical techniques and tests to be applied, an estimate of the average response in one of the treatment groups, the difference between

average responses in two treatment groups which it is clinically important to
have a specified chance (or power) of detecting (assuming it exists) using a test
of statistical significance at some prespecified level. For responses measured on
a continuous scale (such as RTs) we also need an estimate of variation. The
power is usually chosen as 80, 90, or 95%, and the prespecified level of significance at P = 0.05. For further details with explanation in terms of Type I and
Type II errors see Pocock (1983) and Johnson (1989).

As an example I return to a RCT designed to compare the efficacy of two
antiepileptic drugs with a secondary aim of assessing their effects on cognitive
function. We can assume that patients are randomized to one of the two drugs
and then followed-up for a period of 2 years. If we choose a remission period of
1 year as the main measure of response, we then know from previous studies
that about 60% patients will have achieved this by 2 years of follow-up (Elwes
et al. 1984; de Silva et al. 1989). We assume that the times to achieving a period
of 1-year remission in the two groups will be compared using actuarial survival
techniques, and tested statistically by the logrank test. If we require 80% power
to detect an improvement of 15% (that is, 75% patients achieving 1-year
remission by 2 years of follow-up) by this test at the conventional significance
level of 5% (P = 0.05), assuming such a difference exists, then we need a RCT
with at least 140 patients in each group, or a total of 280 patients (Machin &
Campbell 1987). Allowing loss to follow-up of no more than 10%, we must
recruit over 300 patients. Such a sample size immediately suggests a multicenter study if recruitment of patients is to be completed in a relatively short
period of time.

To estimate the sensitivity of such a RCT to detect changes in performance
on a test of cognitive function such as SRT, we need additional information,
which must come either from previous trials in broadly similar patients, or from
studies of test performance. Specifically we need estimates of the variation in
SRT between patients, and of the difference or percentage changes in mean
SRT due to drug effects that we wish to detect. To continue the example, we
can use estimates from our trial with a warning that these are for illustration
only; designers of future studies should ensure that they use estimates pertinent
to the population under study and the tests included in the battery. We assume
that mean RTs in the two drug groups after 2 years of follow-up will be
compared using a standard two-sample t-test on the logarithmically transformed data. The between-patient SD for the SRT estimated from our study is
0.3 msec (on the natural logarithm scale). Reference to the appropriate sample
size tables shows that with 280 patients available for analysis we can detect an
effect size of 0.34 with 80% power at P = 0.05; *effect size* is defined as the
difference between the group means divided by the between-patient SD. So
with group means denoted by M_1 and M_2, and remembering that our data are
logarithmically transformed we get

$$\ln M_1 - \ln M_2 = 0.34 \times 0.3 = 0.102,$$

or M_1/M_2 = 1.11. Here, "ln" denotes natural logarithms (base e). We can therefore detect changes as small as 11% in mean reaction times between the two drug groups, assuming such differences exist. This is equivalent to a change of 54 msec at an average of 500 msec, or of 110 msec at an average of 1 s; changes that are quite small. An increase of 100 msec at an average of 500 msec is equivalent to a change of 20%, or an effect size of just over 0.6 in our example. Eighty percent power of detecting this effect at P = 0.05 can be achieved with just 90 patients. (Further refinements with consequent reduction in sample size may be achieved by analyzing changes from baseline rather than SRT at 2-years' follow-up.) In a multicenter RCT this offers some flexibility in design, either by restricting the computerized tests to just some of the centers, or by stratifying the sample by age so that different age groups can be assessed using different tests. It must be emphasized that such niceties of design require reliable information about the tests themselves.

Conclusion

The design and conduct of randomized clinical trials needs to be as simple and efficient as possible. It is feasible to enter large numbers of patients with epilepsy into clinical trials, to follow most of them over prolonged periods, and consequently to produce a clinically useful result (Medical Research Council Antiepileptic Drug Withdrawal Study Group 1991). When RCTs have more than one outcome of interest and these are of a disparate nature, both the design and the conduct become more complicated. This has been emphasized here in the context of clinical trials designed to undertake comparative assessment of both the efficacy and cognitive side effects of antiepileptic drugs. Some of the problems in the use of computers to assess the latter have been indicated. At present the principal need is for more information about the tests themselves. Until we are in possession of reliable data that indicate the way in which these tests change with respect to age and other characteristics of the populations under investigation, we do not have the means to design clinical trials and other important studies.

References

Altman DG. Comparability of randomized groups. *Statistician*, 1985, 34:125–136.
Altman DG & Bland M. Measurement in medicine in the analysis of method comparison studies. *Statistician*, 1983, 32:307–317.
Altman DG et al. Statistical guidelines for contributors to medical journals. *British Medical Journal*, 1983, 286:1489–1493.

Bland M & Altman DG. Statistical methods for assessing agreement between two methods of clinical measurement. *Lancet*, 1986, i:307-310.

Boissel JP & Klimt CR. (1979). *Multi-center controlled trials: Principles and problems.* Paris: INSERM.

Buyse ME et al. (eds.). (1984). *Cancer clinical trials: Methods and practice.* Oxford: Oxford University Press.

Capildeo R & Orgogozo JM. (eds.). (1988). *Methods in clinical trials in neurology: Vascular and degenerative brain disease.* Basingstoke: Macmillan.

Chinn, S. The assessment of methods of measurement. *Statistics in Medicine*, 1990, 9:351-362.

Corcoran E. Calculating reality. *Scientific American*, 1991, 264:74-83.

Day SJ. Clinical trial numbers and confidence intervals of pre-specified size. *Lancet*, 1988, ii:1427.

de Silva M et al. (1989). A prospective randomized comparative monotherapy clinical trial in childhood epilepsy. In: D Chadwick (ed.), *Fourth International Symposium on Sodium Valproate and Epilepsy* (pp. 81-84). London: Royal Society of Medicine Services.

Dixon WJ. (ed.). (1988). *BMDP statistical software manual* (vol. 2). Berkeley: University of California Press.

Elwes RDC et al. The prognosis for seizure control in newly diagnosed epilepsy. *New England Journal of Medicine*, 1984, 311:944-947.

Friedman LM, Furberg CD & DeMets DL. (1985). *Fundamentals of clinical trials* (2d ed.). Littleton, MA: PSG Publishing Co., Inc.

Gardner MJ & Altman DG. (eds.). (1989). *Statistics with confidence: Confidence intervals and statistical guidelines.* London: British Medical Journal.

Good CS. (ed.). (1976). *The principles and practice of clinical trials.* Edinburgh: Churchill Livingstone.

Health and Safety Executive. Visual Display Units. HMSO, 1983.

Health and Safety Executive. Working with VDU's. HSE, 1986.

Johnson AL. (1984). Statistical aspects of anticonvulsant trials. In: SD Shorvon & GFB Birdwood (eds.), *Rational approaches to anticonvulsant drug therapy* (pp. 13-21). Bern: Hans Huber.

Johnson AL. (1989). Methodology of clinical trials in psychiatry. In: C Freeman & P Tyrer (eds.), *Research methods in psychiatry: A beginner's guide* (pp. 12-45). London: Royal College of Psychiatrists.

Johnson, FN & Johnson S. (eds.). (1977). *Clinical trials.* Oxford: Blackwell.

Jones B & Kenward MG. (1989). *Design and analysis of cross-over trials.* London: Chapman Hall.

Machin D & Campbell MJ. (1987). *Statistical tables for the design of clinical trials.* Oxford: Blackwell.

Medical Research Council Antiepileptic Drug Withdrawal Study Group. (1991). A randomized study of antiepileptic drug withdrawal in patients in remission. *Lancet*, 1991, 337:1175-1180.

Meinert CL. (1986). *Clinical trials: Design, conduct and analysis.* New York: OUP.

Peto R et al. Design and analysis of randomized clinical trials requiring prolonged observation of each patient. I: Introduction and design. *British Journal of Cancer*, 1976, 34:585-612.

Peto R et al. Design and analysis of randomized clinical trials requiring prolonged observation of each patient. II: Analysis and examples. *British Journal of Cancer*, 1977, 35:1–39.

Pocock SJ. (1983). *Clinical trials: A practical approach*. Chichester: Wiley.

Rotmensz N, Vantongelen K & Renard J. (eds.). (1989). *Data management and clinical trials*. Amsterdam: Elsevier.

Schwartz D, Flamant R & Lellouch J. (1980). *Clinical trials* (trans: MRJ Healy). New York: Academic Press.

Shapiro SH & Louis TA. (eds.). (1983). *Clinical trials: Issues and approaches*. Basle: Dekker.

Simpson et al. The cognitive drug research computerized assessment system for demented patients: A validation study. *International Journal of Geriatric Psychiatry*, 1991, 6:95–102.

Spriet A & Simon P. (1985). *Methodology of clinical drug trials*. Basle: Karger.

Sternberg S. High-speed scanning in human memory. *Science*, 1966, 153:652–654.

Tygstrup N, Lachin JM & Juhl E. (1982). *The randomized clinical trial and therapeutic decisions*. New York: Dekker.

Wesnes K et al. A double-blind placebo-controlled trial of Tanakan in the treatment of idiopathic cognitive impairment in the elderly. *Human Psychopharmacology*, 1987, 2:159–169.

Workshop on Methods for Longitudinal Data Analysis in Epidemiological and Clinical Studies. *Statistics in Medicine*, 1988, 7:1–362.

—————— **10** ——————

Workshop
Assessing Cognitive Function
in Patients with Epilepsy

M.D. Lezak
Department of Neurology, School of Medicine
Oregon Health Sciences University

Discussion

Selecting Tests to Evaluate Behavioral Effects of Anticonvulsant Medications

I propose to play devil's advocate regarding extensive use of computers in the assessment of drug effects on the cognitive functioning of epileptic patients. But first, as context for my recommendations—and reservations—I would like to suggest how one might think about developing a program for assessing medication effects on cognition. Although many of these suggestions may seem obvious, the most obvious requirements are not infrequently overlooked and thus need restating.

1. In planning any assessment program the two salient questions are: What to assess? and How to assess? Answers differ according to the nature of the patients' problems and their capacities and limitations; and to practical considerations related to both patient capacities, and to the objective circumstances under which the assessment must take place.

a. What to Assess?

The cognitive function examination of epileptic patients generally should cover 5 major performance areas:

(1) That slowing of both mental processing and motor response occurs with anticonvulsant medications has been well demonstrated (e.g., Trimble & Thompson 1986). Thus measurement of performance speed should be a necessary component of this assessment program.

(2) Because epilepsy is a condition of *disordered attention*, one contribution of anticonvulsant medication should be the amelioration of the accompanying attentional disorder(s). The medication effects need to be studied in terms of each major dimension of attention including (a) *auditory span*, which, when reduced, has direct negative consequences for communication efficiency and, indirectly, contributes to social dysfunction; (b) the capacity for *concentration* and *warding off distractions*, which, when compromised, makes it difficult for the patient to perform activities that take place with groups, in noisy situations, and under competing conditions (such as trying to keep up with two conversations at a time, follow a recipe with a TV program in the background, or monitor and correct as needed one's ongoing performance); (c) *mental tracking*, which, when intact, maintains the consistency and integrity of such complex activities as mental arithmetic or holding onto the thread of a branched story or series of steps toward a goal; and (d) the ability to *shift* one's attention rapidly and appropriately (see Sohlberg & Mateer 1989). Each of these aspects of attention can be vulnerable either to the epileptic condition or to medication effects that slow mental processing; or these may improve when medication effects are therapeutic.

(3) *Memory* complaints are common among epileptic patients. Many of these "memory" problems are actually due to such attentional defects as a short auditory span and distractibility that reduce the amount of information initially registered, thus giving the impression that these patients did not remember stimuli to which they had obviously been exposed. Yet other memory complaints do relate to retention or retrieval deficits. The presence of memory problems needs to be documented and their nature needs to be sorted out. One might anticipate that those memory problems essentially due to attentional deficits would improve with effective seizure control; those due to structural damage within the memory systems may or may not benefit significantly from anticonvulsant medication.

(4) General knowledge (including language knowledge, such as vocabulary) and practical reasoning and judgment tend to be relatively resilient to the effects of brain damage and to reflect a general mental ability potential that can serve as a within-subject yardstick against which more vulnerable functions can

be evaluated for deficit (Lezak 1983 [3d ed. forthcoming]). Abilities to reason and to demonstrate one's knowledge should not be significantly affected by anticonvulsant medication. Because knowledge and reasoning tests are usually verbal, these can also serve as indicators of significant verbal deficits symptomatic of lateralized damage.

(5) The evaluation of visuospatial and visual recognition abilities provides the other half of the evaluation for lateralized cognitive disorders.

In addition to cognitive functions, executive functions, emotional status, and social competence should be reviewed.

Executive functions—the abilities to initiate, plan, and carry out goal-directed and practically self-serving activities—are essential for independent social functioning; the regulatory functions of self-monitoring and self-correction are necessary for effective performance of activities, including social interactions (Lezak 1982; Shallice 1988). Some aspects of executive dysfunction relate to attentional deficits; others involve defects in highest level integrative systems. Their assessment is usually indirect (noting errors, perseverations, inappropriate responses) on tests of cognitive functions, although some direct methods have been developed.

The examination of *emotional status* and *social competence* should be an important component of a study evaluating anticonvulsant medication effects (Dodrill 1986).

b. *How to Assess?*

This question deals with *test selection* and with the *circumstances of the examination*. The two aspects of the question are sufficiently interdependent in this situation that they can be treated as one. Because this examination is being planned for a drug study with repeated assessments rather than clinical evaluations the chief limitations on test selection are time, minimization of practice effects, and suitability of the same or very similar tests over a wide age range and for a patient population in which sensory or motor deficits may be present at a greater-than-normal rate. Moreover, since a major goal is to study drug effects on specific functions, it becomes important to select tests in which very different functions are not confounded.

A practical *time* limitation is about 2 hours if the examination is to be completed in one session, as epileptic patients generally, and children and older persons in particular, tend to be more than ordinarily prone to fatigue and flagging interest. Additionally, if more than one testing session is required at each time interval, the risk of losing patients to the study is increased. Two hours greatly restricts the amount of testing that can be performed and probably requires that the examination focus predominantly on the most sensitive functions of speed, attention, and memory, with perhaps some quick verbal and visual function screening.

Practice effects can only be minimized, not eliminated. With repeated examinations many patients learn to acquire a set with speeded responses and greater efficiency on the second and later examinations, even when the content of the test changes. These effects can best be minimized in two ways: (1) by giving a second examination shortly after the first under the assumption that most set learning will take place in the first examination; thus, when compared to the second examination, subsequent examinations should show few set effects; and (2) by providing different and equated test contents at each examination session. This latter method, although necessary, can be hard to accomplish because of the need to equate content difficulty. A number of attentional tasks and some memory tests are available that satisfy the criterion of multiple forms with reasonably equated content (e.g., Lewis & Rennick 1979; Moran & Mefford 1959).

Suitability of tests over a wide age range often requires parallel forms, usually one for children and another for adults. Within the adult population, it would seem to be most practical to select those that have proven value with older patients, and always use age-graded evaluation criteria. It is important to note that for elderly persons suitability does not mean simple: tests that are too easy are often relatively insensitive—for example, the attention and concentration items of the Wechsler Memory Scales (Wechsler 1945, 1987). Suitability for persons with sensory or motor disorders requires that visual material be clear, easy to track—that is, unlike the visually overwhelming Minnesota Multiphasic Personality Inventory (MMPI) format (Butcher et al. 1989), and reasonably large but not so large that scanning is required to take in single words. All manual responses should be limited to one hand.

The problem of *confounded* test material is minimal in tests of reaction time and in many attentional tests. Confounded functions are an essential part of memory tests that must use verbal or visual material. However, in order to interpret the findings, it is important that they are as little confounded as possible: for example, a test of rote verbal learning—which should probably be included—should not be confounded with a conceptual component if the information that is wanted is whether the medication in question affects rote learning and free recall. Many popular visuoperceptual and constructional tests are timed (e.g., Picture Completion, Picture Arrangement, Block Design, and Object Assembly of the WAIS-R), confounding response speed with the functions of interest. IQ scores and other summation scores such as an "Impairment Index" are quintessential examples of confounded and neuropsychologically meaningless test scores (Lezak 1988). To ascertain drug effects on visuoperceptual and constructional abilities, use of such timed tests must be avoided, or performances scored without regard to time to completion.

2. "Let the punishment fit the crime," is the call in Gilbert and Sullivan's *Mikado*. While tests should not be considered punishments, the principle of best fit holds for neuropsychological assessment as well as for crime. For some functions, computerized assessment is ideal; for many others, it is inappropriate.

Most of the problems posed by computerized assessment have to do with various limitations presented by the subjects.

(1) *Sustaining interest.* Both very young and very old persons may be unable to sustain interest in these procedures, particularly if they are lengthy and have monotonous content; yet many computerized test programs need to continue for more than 5 or 10 minutes to obtain an adequate sample of responses. Mentally dull persons, who will be more than normally represented in the population of epileptic patients, are also less likely to be able to keep sufficiently interested for adequate performance.

(2) *Maintaining attentiveness.* On any computerized test other than those examining concentration and distractibility, keeping distractable persons sufficiently attentive to accomplish the assessment of the function of interest can present a more serious problem than it does in clinical assessments. In clinical assessments, examiners are continuously attentive to the patient's behavior; they can generally stop procedures when the patient is distracted, resuming them after drawing the patient's attention back to the task; or rerun a timed task interrupted by distractibility. When a patient is responding to a computer it becomes much more difficult to determine whether or not inattention rather than inability produced a lapse in performance or some erroneous responses. Even when the patient's computer performance is being constantly monitored, what should the monitor do when the patient seems to have been distracted? Stop the program? Rerun all of it or just the section that was interrupted? What happens then to standardization?

(3) *Acquiring and maintaining an instructional set.* Certainly some epileptic patients have had little or no experience with a computer or even computerized games. Beyond learning how to interact with the computer, subjects must learn how to do a variety of unfamiliar tasks for which instructions may seem confusing. Although learning how to perform should present a problem for only a few patients, loss of or confusion about an instructional set during a test run is more likely to occur. This problem shows up readily on Wechsler's Picture Completion and Similarities tests: In the former, patients who do not retain a set well begin to search for what they think are mistakes in the pictures; in the latter, they begin to give differences rather than similarities. In clinical examinations the examiner observes the slip in set immediately and can correct it without violating standardization. On a computerized test, the shift in set would show up in errors, but the nature of these errors is never clarified, and the lowered score would be misinterpreted.

(4) *Timing.* Sensory and motor deficits can increase response times and skew test data. Scores on timed tasks obtained by patients with visual limitations or motor slowing should be kept out of the general data pool.

In addition to these problems inherent in the patients, is the *loss of qualitative data*. Computerized testing can severely restrict the examiner's ability to observe what is often the most theoretically interesting and practically relevant behavior: *how* a patient performs. This include aspects of performance such as initiating activities (e.g., spontaneously turning pages, picking up test material), self-monitoring and self-correction, perseverations, confabulatory tendencies, development and maintenance of strategies, planfulness, and impulsivity. Although the presence or absence of some of these performance qualities will be registered as correct or erroneous responses by the computer, the most significant variables contributing to the errors—or good responses—will remain obscured.

One other limitation posed by computers is *administration flexibility.* This may or may not be a consideration in a drug study. However, a wider sample of patients can be obtained if all the test material can be put in the front seat of a car and carried for 100 meters by a woman weighing 50 kgs.

In determining whether or not to use computerized tests it is important, in each instance, to ask: Do the benefits outweigh the problems inherent in computerized assessment?

(1) Computers are much more suited to the assessment of *response speed* than are examiners with stopwatches.

(2) Aspects of *attention* that can be best examined by means of computerized tests include sustained attention (continous performance-type tests), attention as measured by simple and complex reaction time tasks (although here motor components of response speed can contribute a significant confound, which may make interpretation of findings difficult), and visual span (how many items can be encompassed at once). Posner (1988) has demonstrated the effectiveness of computerized assessment in the examination of attentional shift. Distractibility, too, lends itself to computerized testing, although Dodrill's (1978) paper-and-pencil Stroop format has proven invaluable in the examination of epileptic patients' ability to withstand a strong distraction. Mental tracking is usually examined by serial subtractions and other sequential mental operations, and the Paced Auditory Serial Addition Test (PASAT) (Gronwall & Sampson 1974). Other mental tracking tests are available that are less frustrating for the patient and have a wider difficulty range (and therefore greater sensitivity) than the PASAT, and are also available on tape cassettes satisfying standardization requirements (e.g., Weber 1988).

(3) Although many clever computerized tests of memory and learning have been developed, the problems of sustaining interest, and maintaining attention

and set can outweigh considerations of ease of administration, scoring, and compiling data. An adequate and relevant assessment of memory will examine retrieval efficiency by providing the means to distinguish between recall and recognition, the former indicating how much can be retrieved spontaneously, the latter indicating how much was actually stored. This should be done for both rote and meaningful (e.g., story) learning. Moreover, qualitative aspects of the memory performance should be taken into account, and can be readily handled as examination data. For example, on a test of word list learning, repetitions offer evidence of impaired mental tracking, intrusions suggest confabulatory tendencies; both types of error can be tallied. Computerization of tests assessing recognition, both visual and verbal, is more feasible than when recall is required because, although the problems inherent to computerized testing remain, the nature of the recognition task greatly reduces the likelihood of loss of qualitative information.

(4) If a screen for verbal, visuoperceptual, and visuoconstructional functions is included, use of familiar traditional techniques would seem to be advisable because these data can be interpreted readily by both study participants and clinicians to whom study findings are conveyed. Some available and well-known tests are in paper-and-pencil format and are relatively easy to administer. I like to include some paper-and-pencil tests because of the richness of preserved qualitative information. Nontraditional scoring will have to be worked out for timed tests: I typically give two scores when items are completed successfully outside of time limits, one following standard practice, one giving credit to all completed items.

The assessment of emotional status in a research program is usually done with paper-and-pencil inventories. If the instruments used are reasonably short, they could be administered on a computer although again the trade-off would be shortened data handling time against the problems of interest, attention, and set discussed above.

References

Butcher JN, Dahlstrom WG, Graham JR et al. (1989). *Manual for the restandardized Minnesota Multiphasic Personality Inventory: MMPI-2*. Minneapolis: University of Minnesota Press.

Dodrill CB. A neuropsychological battery for epilepsy. *Epilepsia*, 1978, 19:611-623.

Dodrill CB. (1986). Psychosocial consequences of epilepsy. In: SB Filskov & TJ Boll (eds.), *Handbook of clinical neuropsychology* (vol. 2) (pp. 338-363). New York: John Wiley & Sons.

Gronwall DMA & Sampson H. (1974). *The psychological effects of concussion*. New Zealand: Auckland University Press/Oxford University Press.

Lewis RF & Rennick PM. (1979). *Manual for the Repeatable Cognitive-Perceptual Motor Battery*. Grosse Pointe Park, MI: Axon Publishing Co.

Lezak MD. The problem of assessing executive functions. *International Journal of Psychology*, 1982, 17:281-297.

Lezak MD. (1983). *Neuropsychological assessment* (2d ed., 3d ed. forthcoming). New York: Oxford University Press.

Lezak MD. IQ: R.I.P. *Journal of Clinical and Experimental Neuropsychology*, 1988, 10:351-361.

Moran LJ & Mefferd RB Jr. Repetitive psychometric measurements. *Psychological Reports*, 1959, 5:269-275.

Posner MI. (1988). Structures and functions of selective attention. In: TJ Boll & BK Bryant (eds.), *Clinical neuropsychology and brain function: Research, measurement, and practice*. Washington, DC: American Psychological Association.

Shallice T. (1988). *From neuropsychology to mental structure*. New York: Cambridge University Press.

Sohlberg MM & Mateer CA. (1989). *Introduction to cognitive rehabilitation*. New York: Guilford.

Trimble MR & Thompson PJ. (1986). Neuropsychological aspects of epilepsy. In: I Grant & KM Adams (eds.), *Neuropsychological assessment of neuropsychiatric disorders* (pp. 321-346). New York: Oxford University Press.

Weber, AM. A new clinical measure of attention: The Attentional Capacity Test. *Neuropsychology*, 1988, 2:59-71.

Wechsler D. A standardized memory scale for clinical use. *The Journal of Psychology*, 1945, 19:87-95.

Wechsler D (1974). *WISC-R manual. Wechsler Intelligence Scale for Children—revised.* New York: Psychological Corporation.

Wechsler D. (1981). *WAIS—R manual.* New York: Psychological Corporation.

Wechsler D. (1987). *Wechsler Memory Scale-revised. Manual.* San Antonio, TX: Psychological Corporation.

Test Selection and Design for Antiepileptic Drug Neurocognitive Monitoring

Marcel Kinsbourne

Behavioral Neurology Unit, Sargent College of Allied Health Professions
Boston, Massachusetts

Controlled monitoring of neuropsychological performance is an essential supplement to the collection of subjective reports about the side effects of antiepileptic agents. This is particularly important in view of the large number of new and sometimes novel compounds now entering the market (Brodie & Porter 1990). When monitoring an antiepileptic agent for neuropsychological side effects, it is neither efficient nor economical simply to use a general-purpose neuropsychological test battery. Rather, test selection and, where necessary, test design, should be based on a model of the type of disturbances to be anticipated if an antiepileptic agent has a negative effect on neuropsychological functioning. This is primarily so that one should not overlook potentially relevant domains. Next, that when tapping a domain that should be included one uses sensitive tests within that domain. And, finally, so as not to encumber the test repertoire with useless instruments, particularly when time is of the essence. Time is particularly critical when repeated testing is needed to compare anticonvulsants with each other or with placebo, or to monitor anticonvulsant effects over time and across diverse dose levels. I am going to attempt such a mode. It is a fairly simple one, based on some rather simplistic concepts of brain organization.

The cortical mantle of gray matter is responsible for information processing of a categorical nature. Each part ("module") of the network is specialized to generate differently patterned neuronal discharges, which contribute toward the implementation of different types of processing. In contrast, the executive functions are implemented by functionally bidirectional cortico–cortical connections, including the forebrain commissure and loops between cortex and brain stem. These control functions are not responsible for the detailed computing of input and decision. They subserve selection, to determine behavioral precedence; what to do first, what to do right away, what to restrain onself from doing, in what sequence to act to implement a plan. These control functions especially involve the perfrontal lobes, and are mostly mediated by the monoamines, dopamine, norepinephrine, and serotonin (Goldman-Rakic 1987). I assume that when a generalized noxious influence impairs a brain function by means of neurotoxic effects, it will put monoamine production at risk, rather than the computing processes that are localized in modules in various parts of the cerebral mantle. That is why there appears to be little need for specific verbal or spatial or other categorical testing. Specifically, at least some of the anticonvulsants have a GABA-mediated inhibitory effect (Macdonald & Meldrum 1989). They therefore suppress activity in dopamine-, norepinephrine-, and serotonin-mediated circuitry. What might we expect behaviorally from underactivity in these three types of circuits?

What might result from underproduction of *dopamine*, specifically in the mesolimbic orbitofrontal projection? This projection subserves incentive motivation. In practical terms, whereas those who lack incentive motivation remain perfectly capable of meeting their immediate needs and reaction to salient circumstances, they will not do well at anything for which the consequence is delayed, which is taxing, in terms of mental effort, or to which a more salient or familiar alternative response is available.

Inattention, as a consequence of deficient dopamine in the mesolimbic-orbitofrontal projection, can take the form either of withdrawing attention from the situation or of arriving at a premature response. Further, the inattention will be most marked where attending requires an amount of mental effort that is experienced as aversive. A basic distinction exists between two kinds of attention: effortful and effortless. Both are at risk, and both should be measured. Effortful attention in particular is a promising discriminator. In our work with hyperactive (attention-deficient) children, who appear to be deficient in dopamine production, the most sensitive discriminator is not a task such as the Continuous Performance Test (CPT) (see Aman this volume), which though easy is boring—although that does discriminate—but a task such as paired associate learning, which can be made very difficult by choosing unrelated stimulus and response pairs, associating which calls for sustained mental effort.

Impulsivity is a second, though not unrelated, consequence, of deficiency in dopamine. A third is impairment in planning and organization. A fourth consequence, if the deficit is extensive enough, and also implicates the nigrostriatal dopaminergic projection, might be motor slowing (which is prominent among behavioral effects of some anticonvulsants; e.g., Dodrill [1975]).

In her discussion, Lezak (this volume) lists several disadvantages of computerized testing, all of which can be avoided if an observer is present during the testing. Anyone who thinks that they can place an impulsive person or a child in front of a computer and leave them unattended is deluded. I always assume that there is a person attending the child who works at the computer.

Norepinephrine is involved in reaction to novelty; so the ability to notice novel or distinctive aspects of a context is impaired when norepinephrine is deficient. This compromises episodic memory (memory for events), which relies on contextual labeling. People with low norepinephrine production, such as Korsakoff amnesics, have great trouble with contextual labeling of events to be remembered. (Low acetylcholine production is an additional cause of memory problems with GABAergic drugs.) Also, in terms of personality and mood, people with low norepinephrine are subdued, depressed, internally distracted, spacey— a variety of description familiar in children with attention-deficit disorder without hyperactivity. Mental slowing, slowing of responses, is also to be expected if norepinephrine activity is much depressed.

Finally, the level of *serotonin* influences how we evaluate our personal circumstances. The "glass is half-full" if serotonin is high. It is "half-empty" if serotonin production is low. A person with very low serotonin levels is irritable, discontented, complaining, and impulsive in their responding. That person's "reactive" depression is different from the "endogenous" depression in patients with low norepinephrine. The latter patients are inert and unreactive. These mood factors need to be evaluated and can be (by a variety of psychiatric checklists and questionnaires that are plentifully used in other fields) suitably applied to this field, for example, the Child Behavior Checklist (Miles et al. 1988).

Newer antiepileptic agents may be NMDA receptor antagonists, and thus also impair memory.

The administration of tests of attention, impulse control, memory and motor control here recommended corresponds well with existing knowledge of the behavioral side effects of anticonvulsants, as summarized in the preceding chapters of this book. Memory and motor speed have been much emphasized; inattention and impulsivity have been remarked upon, but less often measured. Given tests that tap the anticipated neurotransmitter insufficiency, what properties must such tests have to be useful for monitoring? Whatever test is used, if one is going to use it to monitor changing states, one has to have an initial familiarization and practice session. One cannot use the data of the first session, wasteful though that might appear to be, because it is a massive source of uncontrolled variance generated while a child gets used to the situation, the staff, and overcomes his or her reluctance to be there in the first place.

One needs a task that can be given many times at the same level of difficulty, not just two or three times, but eight, or ten or twelve times (as when we monitor the stimulant response of hyperactive children). Any task that does not lend itself to an almost indefinite number of equally difficult alternative forms is not a good choice for monitoring anticonvulsant effects on cognition. It may be a good choice for diagnostic work, but monitoring is a different enterprise. Here the computer has a great advantage. It can shuffle the items and produce an alternate form at each test session. (Other advantages are the precise timing, and the avoidance of experimenter effects, which are particularly troublesome when attention is being tested.)

Second, one also has to be sure that the alternate form will give zero transfer. There must be no practice effects, which give positive transfer, so that one does better the second time than the first time, on equally difficult material. Nor must one have retroactive inhibition effects, which give negative transfer. When one develops a test one must be able to show that it can be given a number of times to normal children or adults without any statistically significant main effect of the order of sessions. Otherwise one confuses oneself by trying to guess how much effect was practice, how much was drug-level related. Obviously that requirement restricts the range of tests one can use because there are certain tests that are difficult to envisage in terms of multiple alternative equally difficult forms.

The third matter to attend to is, how long the test takes. How long does a test normally take? If the answer is: as long as its designer wanted it to, this is common but not a good enough reason. A test should take long enough so that if it were any longer one would not learn substantially more. How does one determine that? By giving it for a long time, for half an hour or an hour and then by doing a time series analysis so as to discover how well the scores of the initial segments of the test correlate with the total score. If one finds a 0.9 correlation between the core after 5 min and the score after 30 min, one does not have to continue the test for 30 min.

The format of the test should also be amenable to the computation of variability; that is, the successive time segments have to be comparable. This is not true for a traditional learning test administered across multiple trials. Given a word list over and over again, one cannot compare the amount learned in the first minute, second, and third minute because the task keeps changing as some words are learned, some are overlearned, and some are not as yet learned. We have designed the continuous paired associate learning test (C-PALT), in a way such that consecutive epochs are comparable and can be used to compute performance variability (see below).

The coefficient of variation is the statistic that represents variability independent of mean performance. Variability is of the essence in attention problems. The unpredictability of ADHD behavior is notorious. This is because in the absence of dopamine-supported planfulness, behavior is at the beck and call of moment-to-moment change in the environment. When we construct dose-response and time-response curves for stimulant effects in hyperactive children, if we plot changes in variability we obtain curves that distinguish dose levels to a degree that is as clear cut as when we plot means. Indeed, changes in coefficient of variation are the more informative because being performance-free, these can be used to compare young and older children, and bright and slow people by means of the same statistic (Kinsbourne 1990).

It is also necessary to have an effective reinforcement system for performing the test. For example, when testing an adult male patient who has a local brain lesion, neuropsychologists tend to assume that the person is imbued with the Protestant ethic. Any problem that he has in performing a task is assumed to be because he really cannot do it. He is trying as hard as the clinician would try in the same situation. If the individual is not, the clinician nags him until he does. But that is not going to work with children, let alone with mentally disturbed children, any more than it does with mentally retarded children, as behavioral psychologists know. The child has to know what is in it for him to do that work, and has to be reinforced in a way appropriate to that child, giving him something he wants. Otherwise a source of variability remains that counfounds the data.

Having made this wish list of what a monitoring task should be like, I shall mention some of the ways in which we have resolved comparable problems with respect to our attention-deficit disorder (ADD) children and our computerized monitoring tasks (Kinsbourne 1990). For maintaining attention, we have made our effortful C-PALT as arid as possible so as to inhibit interest as well as preclude the child from discovering a strategy in the course of the testing. The stimuli are sets of three consonants, and the responses are digits. The computer begins by presenting three consonants and then the digit response. Next the screen shows just the consonants and the subject keys in the digit response, whereupon another set of consonants appears, followed by the response, and so on. The task is programmed in a way such that one can analyze it to compare learning ability within successive epochs. We run the test for half an hour, then break the data down into 3-min segments, and plot the individual's variability in learning across 10 data points. From these we can derive a coefficient of variation.

Any task of attention always tests something in addition to attention. One should therefore not confine oneself to any one task of attention in case one is dealing with somebody whose specific ability, for instance in verbal learning, given verbal paired associates, is compromised, and confounds the measurement with floor effects. Nonetheless, the PALT turns out to be our most sensitive index for drug effects. It is a good instrument for discovering not only which attention-deficit individuals respond favorably to stimulant medication, but also what is the most beneficial dose level.

We have developed another task that calls for intense maintained attention and is effortful. Whereas in the paired associate task the effort is invested in maintaining rehearsing, thinking back, in our *pursuit task* the effort is all in the moment-to-moment attending. A circle is exhibited on the computer screen, and the subject manipulates the mouse to keep a cursor inside the circle. The circle moves about unpredictably at a considerable rate. The subject has to try very hard to maintain continuous attention, and what he or she is trying very hard to do has not, in the least bit, been made interesting.

For monitoring relatively effortless attention there are many suitable continuous performance tasks (CPTs) in which subjects are required to be alert consistently over significant time periods for relatively infrequent target stimuli. We use one in which a string of letters is exposed at each trial, *Letter Detection*. When a letter is repeated in the string the subject depresses the response button. What is special about this CPT, is that we have verified zero transfer across sessions. Maybe other existing CPTs would also show zero transfer if tested for this attribute.

I distinguish between two kinds of impulsivity: perceptual and motor. We evaluate perceptual impulsivity by means of our *Flag Test*. Imagine an incoming military aircraft. One of yours or one of theirs? If it is one of yours it carries your code. If it is one of theirs it has a code that differs in one or more details. As the incoming airplane approaches, slowly the identifying symbols come into view. They are faint at first and then they become clearer and clearer. The longer you wait the more sure you are of the decision: yes, this is ours; or no, it is the other side's. However, there is an on-secreen number representing credits, starting from 1000, that is rapidly diminishing while you think. So you are in a high-drive state. To test impulsivity it is necessary to induce a high-drive state. Otherwise one may merely be eliciting carelessness or noncompliance, which are different. Thus there is the pull to be careful and not make a mistake, losing all 1000 points, and penalized as well. At the same time you try to be as quick as you can because the points are dwindling away. People with deficient attention are known to be particularly sensitive to "response cost," which is what this is. So our Flag Test is designed to measure perceptual impulsivity or impulsive decision making; making hasty decisions before the information is complete enough.

We also have a motor impulsivity test, which we call the *Delayed Bomb*. As in the well-known procedure called Differential Reinforcement for Low Rates of Responding (DRL) the response is predetermined, but one has to wait a certain period of time or one does not get the reinforcement. A surface at the foot of the screen represents where you live (Earth), and a bomb is seen to be dropping toward it. The mouse controls a cursor that can disarm the bomb and save Earth. But this only works after a little white light appears momentarily in the bomb. If you are not watching, Earth will not be saved. If the response is in time, the bomb blows up rather gratifyingly. So, here we evaluate the ability to restrain a motor response. There is no decisional uncertainty; it is purely a matter of timing.

Organization and planning are attributes for which existing tests are the least adequate. In our *Code Test*, again a bomb is dropping onto a surface at the foot of the screen. One can disarm it by finding the right code. In the most difficult condition, there is a 2 × 4 matrix of circles. Only one combination of these locations constitutes the code to disarm the bomb. You have no idea what it is. You try one, arbitrarily. The bomb continues to drop and blows up your house. After having tried four or five of these combinations without success, one wonders: Which ones have I not yet tried? Does the subject devise a strategy, so that he or she can systematically keep track?

There are innumerable memory tests. The ones we have developed meet the aforementioned criteria. One is for *remembering locations*. The computer presents a number of randomly arranged rectangles, two of which are blackened in. After a period of time it shows the same pattern, but without any rectangles blackened. The subject has to indicate the two circles that were previously blackened in. Sometimes the computer makes the subject wait a long time while holding those target locations in mind. This introduces the pertinent mental effort or concentration component. For *object memory* we have adapted an existing test, delayed recognition span. Pictures of objects appear on the screen. On each successive trial the same objects appear as before, plus a new one (all randomized in position). The subject indicates each new one. He or she remembers which ones had previously appeared, up to the point at which the limit of his or her memory span is reached and then selects an old one by mistake.

Finally, we measure alertness by means of *serial reaction times*. One needs a reaction time task that is going to generate a plateau of performance soon, so that the test is not unduly time consuming. In the test that we use, there are four squares in a row on the CRT. As a dot appears in a square the subject superimposes the cursor controlled by a mouse. As soon as he or she has done this, a dot appears in another square, and so on.

The computer tallies the total latency of response. Built in is a segment where, unknown to the subjects, the pattern becomes predictable in that it repeats itself over 10 trials. This is usually not even recognized by the subject. Nonetheless reaction times speed up. This gives an estimate of the ability to automatize.

Controls are useful for determining the comparative sensitivity of various tests, as determined by discriminant analysis. When there is a decline in performance on a task on a given drug, what does this actually mean in real-life circumstances? Is the change potentially important? The distribution of control values will tell one whether the slippage due to the medication is minor or major. This helps decide where to concentrate subsequent neuropsychological efforts.

In conclusion, it is probably not the best strategy to use an existing neuropsychological battery if designed for other purposes. It is preferable to be eclectic, and to choose those tasks which appear most likely to be sensitive to what one is looking for. Otherwise one might conclude that a drug really has no impact on cognitive processes, when in fact the tests were insensitive.

Whether or not they are preferable for diagnostic testing, computerized procedures are clearly better suited to monitoring performance change by repeated testing. Unlike the human tester, the computer always retests in the same way, without delivering irrelevant cues. Alternate forms are easily generated, latencies are measured, and the results computed and printed out without delay. Some computers are now easily portable, so that the location of the test is not an issue. The clinician is not replaced or redundant, but stays with the patient during the test, is freed to make concurrent behavioral observations, and verifies the patient's task orientation. Human resources are not replaced, but optimized.

References

Brodie MJ & Porter RJ. New and potential anticonvulsants. *Lancet*, 1990, 336: 425–426.

Dodrill CB. Diphenylhydantoin serum levels, toxicity and neuropsychological performance in patients with epilepsy. *Epilepsia*, 1975, 16:593–600.

Goldman-Rakic PS. Development of cortical circuitry and cognitive function. *Child Development*, 1987, 58:601–622.

Kinsbourne M. (1990). Testing models for attention deficit hyperactivity disorder in the behavioral laboratory. In: M Kinsbourne & CK Conners (eds.), *Diagnosis and treatment of attention deficit disorder* (pp. 51–70). Munich: MMW Press.

Macdonald RL & Meldrum BS. (1989). Principles of anti-epileptic drug action. In: R Levy, R Mattson, BS Meldrum et al. (eds.), *Antiepileptic drugs* (3d ed.) (pp. 59–83). New York: Raven Press.

Miles MV, Tennison MB & Greenwood RS. (1988). Assessment of antiepileptic drug effects on child behavior using the child behavior checklist. *Journal of Epilepsy*, 1988, 1:209–213.

───────── **12** ─────────

Neuropsychological Assessment of Development Compounds

Beat Hiltbrunner
Ciba-Geigy Limited
Basel, Switzerland

The efficacy of first-line anticonvulsant medications in the treatment of generalized tonic–clonic epilepsy, such as phenytoin, phenobarbitone, carbamazepine and valproate, varies little (Brodie 1990). The deleterious effects of barbiturates on behavior and cognitive function have frequently been emphasized and used to justify the prescription of the newer anticonvulsant compounds (Trimble 1987). However, the debate on the methodology to establish the comparative frequency and severity of side effects of various antiepileptic compounds has not abated.

Many factors influence the mental performance of patients with epilepsy. The brain lesion that underlies the epileptic seizures; the degree of disturbed electrophysiological activity of the brain; social, cultural, and educational problems stand out as factors that affect the performance of patients in cognitive testing. As compared to the factors mentioned above, antiepileptic medications probably contribute rather little to the impairment of cognitive function. The effects of anticonvulsants on cognitive function are difficult to assess. Furthermore, the acute side effects of anticonvulsants may differ from those that arise during long-term treatment, and therefore have different implications for the treatment of patients. Precautions can be taken to protect the patient during the start-up phase of therapy. The long-term

— 171 —

effects of phenytoin treatment on memory are more difficult to avoid. Keeping the patient on the lowest plasma concentration that provides relief from epileptic seizures is the most obvious such attempt. Given such examples, it is not surprising that the health authorities now require that the magnitude of short- and long-term treatment effects on cognitive function and mood be assessed for the purpose of registering new anticonvulsant medications.

The scope and contents of a program to assess drug effects on cognitive function must reflect a clear understanding of how new compounds are developed. The primary goal is to prove that the new compound is efficacious and safe in its main indication. The risk-to-benefit ratio of a proposed new treatment must be demonstrated to be favorable. A comprehensive development program is necessary to meet these requirements. In phase I, healthy adult volunteers are administered the putative new medication, in acute single and multidose studies, to determine its pharmacokinetic and pharmacodynamic properties. In phase IIa several doses of the new compound are given to a small number of patients with epilepsy, again to evaluate its pharmacokinetics, safety, and tolerability. The goal of phase IIb is to establish effective dose ranges in the primary epilepsy indication. Phase III finally enables a more precise definition of the effective treatment regimen and indications of the new compound. This complex and time-consuming process advances in discrete stages demarcated by a review of newly acquired data before each next development phase is initiated. The documentation on all investigations, together with an expert report that reviews, summarizes, and interprets the essential data of the complete development program, are submitted to the health authorities. The data on the effects on cognitive function are an integral part of the registration dossier (CMPM Working Party 1989).

The methodology of clinical trials to assess anticonvulsant effects on cognitive function has greatly advanced in recent years. Some investigators subscribe to ad hoc compositions of individual tests to assess specific hypotheses, others to neuropsychological batteries that provide information on a wide variety of cognitive abilities (see Lezak, this volume). The selection of specific tests depends on the goal of the clinical trial, the format of testing, the number of sessions and the frequency with which these are to be repeated and the availability of alternate test forms (see Kinsbourne, this volume). Traditional neuropsychological testing consists of questionnaires and paper-and-pencil tests. Over the past 10 years, computerized tests have been added and are rapidly becoming accepted and even irreplaceable. But information on their reliability and validity is scanty. Their major strength is that repeated testing is made possible by the easy generation of alternate formats. Further, computerized tests can easily be adapted to the patients' level of mental ability by preselecting the presentation rate, time available for response, interstimulus interval, and test duration. As described in previous chapters, computerized testing does not diminish the need for the support of competent psychologists who ensure that the patients understand the test requirements and who observe them during testing. The advantages and disadvantages of both computerized and traditional techniques have been reviewed in previous chapters. As part of a drug development program, computerized neuropsychological tests have obvious potential advantages in terms of standardization of test application in multicenter studies and in facility of data collection.

Piloting of neuropsychological tests for an anticonvulsant medication development program is needed in phase I before more extensive patient populations are studied. It can be debated whether cognitive function assessments of healthy volunteers are likely to contribute importantly to understanding the drug's effects on the epileptic target population. Obviously, if a new anticonvulsant medication induces cognitive deficits in healthy volunteers, its application to epileptic patients requires particular care. Since the initial studies are acute single- and multiple-dose investigations, piloting of the neuropsychological test battery cannot be completed during this phase. Certain acute medication effects may occur in healthy individuals but not in patients with epilepsy. With continued treatment, other acute toxic effects may abate rapidly and be of no real-life significance. The choice of neuropsychological tests should therefore ideally be based on knowledge of the pharmacological effects of the new compound. In view of the length of time that it takes to develop new antiepileptic compounds, it is of paramount importance to select sensitive neuropsychological tests from the start of the clinical development program. An important detrimental neuropsychological effect of a new compound may abort its development. Failing to detect such an effect in time, or failing to compare a profile of cognitive side effects of a new compound to that of marketed medications, may prove expensive for the developer if the registration dossier is for this reason rejected by the health authority. In order to obtain a broad overview of the effects of a new compound, behavior, mood, and emotional states should be investigated as well.

In children, scholastic achievement represents a central concern as a positive effect of cognitive impairments caused by anticonvulsant medication (see Aman, this volume). Treatment is only one—and probably the least important—determinant of educational achievement in children with epilepsy. Other factors, such as frequency of missed classes due to intercurrent epileptic seizures, the nature of the underlying brain pathology, and the psychosocial milieu influence the quality and quantity of educational progress. When the effects of anticonvulsant medication on mental performance in children are studied, these confounding factors need to be assessed and taken into account. A number of standardized and graded scholastic achievement tests exist that are suitable for repeated testing of children educated in most Western educational systems. Neuropsychological tests employed to determine anticonvulsant medication effects need to be sensitive to maturational changes in mental performance and suitable for repeated testing as described in a previous chapter by Marcel Kinsbourne (this volume). The selected tests should also include some that allow a comparison of the new with the marketed compounds.

Cognitive effects of a new anticonvulsant medication may vary according to the plasma drug concentration. In order to study this problem one should know the approximate relationship between dose, plasma drug concentration, efficacy, and tolerance. This information is often only available at the end of the development of a new compound. Plasma-concentration related cognitive impairments additionally may only be detected by particularly sensitive neuropsychological tests.

Among the numerous neuropsychological tests currently employed to study the effects of antiepileptic medication on cognitive function only few meet stringent scientific criteria that justify their use in an antiepileptic medication development program. A bank of standardized, validated neuropsychological tests would assist the pharmaceutical industry in selecting those tests that fit the particular pharmacological profile of a new antiepileptic compound. The workshop participants suggested that both paper-and-pencil and computerized tests ought to be included in a development program. Individual tests were to be selected on empirical and theoretical grounds and fulfill certain quality criteria, including: (1) validity and reliability, (2) availability in parallel forms, (3) demonstrated applicability (e.g., not too time consuming, generalizeable across cultures) to the patient population to be studied, (4) economical demand on equipment resource and staff support, and (5) availability of adequate testing instruction. The spectrum of domains tested as part of a neuropsychological assessment of an antiepileptic development compound should be wide and include: (1) an inventory of subjective complaints, (2) efficacy and toxicity measures, (3) activity of daily living and quality of life measures, (4) sensory-motor function, and (5) psychosocial and scholastic achievement, where applicable.

Computer-driven neuropsychological tests were thought to be preferable for the study of speed and attention, impulse control, and executive functions because they allow precising timing of test parameters (stimulus exposure, response time, item frequency), as discussed above. In multicenter studies, computerized tests should be favored to avoid tester bias and variability in test application. Traditional tests may be used to study learning and memory, judgment, visuospatial function, verbal functions, and mood. In general, however, whenever both a conventional and a computerized test are available, the latter version should be chosen provided its psychometric properties are acceptable. Finally, psychophysiological tests, across several modalities, even including the olfactory, and with respect to several parameters, including temporal discrimination and judgment of duration, are potentially sensitive to medication effects. Some workshop participants advocated a broad screening of neuropsychological functions during the initial pilot studies. Others emphasized that multiple tests in a small number of patients would incur the risk of committing type II errors, on account of lack of statistical power and that test selection should be guided by hypotheses. However, more neuropsychological tests than will subsequently prove to be necessary are likely to be used during this initial phase of testing. Consequently, a reduction to a justifiable minimum of tests is required for larger scale studies. The participants were reluctant to name specific tests that should routinely be used in the initial screening of a new antiepileptic compound. They suggested that such recommendations be based on a review of the literature by a panel of experts in neuropsychological testing. Meta-analyses were recommended to evaluate the sensitivity of certain neuropsychological tests. Collaboration of major centers specializing in neuropsychological testing would strengthen the scientific backing of neuropsychological testing in epilepsy.

References

Brodie MJ. (1990). Established anticonvulsants and treatment of refractory epilepsy. *The Lancet*, Epilepsy; A Lance Review, pp. 20–25.

Trimble MR. Anticonvulsant drugs and cognitive function: A review of the literature. *Epilepsia*, 1987, 28 (suppl. 3):37–45.

CMPM Working Party on Efficacy of Medicinal Product. (1989). Note for Guidance III/3128/88. Medicinal Products for the Treatment of Epileptic Disorders (1990 Revision). Commission of the European Communities.

Absence epilepsy, 128
Ad hoc clinical tests, for the detection of transitory cognitive impairment, 129
Adaptive testing, 41
Anticonvulsant medications, and neuropsychological function, 13, side effects, 60, 171, possible reduction of pathology with increasing dosage, 120
Antidepressants, effects on neuropsychological assessment, 45
Assessment, of abstract thinking, 38, of perceptual motor speed, 37, of visual perceptual analysis, 37, of visuospatial ability, 37, 157
Attention Deficit Disorder, 121, 167
Attention Deficit-Hyperactivity Disorder (ADHD), 69
Attention, measurement of, 74, 160, medication effects on, 156, disordered, 156
Auditory span, medication effects on, 156
Auditory-Visual (A-V) Integration Task, 72, 78
Automobile braking simulator, 25
Bender Gestalt test, 10, Canter Background Interference Procedure for, 10
Benzodiazepines, effects on neuropsychological assessment, 45
Binary Choice Reaction Test, 54, 63
Bromides, 14
Carbamazapine, 14, 54, effects on psychometric variables in children, 77
Centrencephalic seizures, 7

Chalfont Center for Epilepsy, 4
Childhood epilepsy, 54, and cognitive status, 12
Choice reaction time, 54, 63, 100, 113, 144, for the detection of transitory cognitive impairment, 129
Clinical trials, methodology, 172
Clobazam, 46
Clonazepan, 46
Code Test, 169
Cognitive assessment, traditional, 1, history, 2
Cognitive changes, associated with psychopharmacologic investigations, 45, subtle, 45, mental slowing, 45, 62, 156
Cognitive deterioration, 3
Cognitive dysfunction, and subclinical epileptogenic activity, 112, 113, unawareness of, 56
Cognitive failure, unawareness of, 57
Cognitive performance, effects of spike wave discharges on, 7
Cognitive status, beneficial effects of improved seizure control on, 11
Cognitive-Motor Battery, 79
Complex reaction time tasks, 61
Complex Visual Searching Test (CVST), 54, 63, 64
Computer programming languages, 26
Computer programs, scoring and interpretation, 39
Computer system, selfcontained, 24, driving peripheral equipment, 24, types of hardware systems, 24
Computer-assisted neuro-psychological tests, 110, complications of, 110
Computerized neuropsychological